Praise for *Unavoidably Unsafe for Adults*

"Drs. Geehr and Barke have done it again, but this time for adult vaccines. A must-read."

—Del Bigtree

"Why do adults need vaccines? Are they safe? Do they work and for how long? Adults all over the world are asking these questions with the rapidly expanding array of products offered to prevent infections. With clarity, Drs. Geehr and Barke peel back the burgeoning adult immunization schedule and critique medical necessity, clinical indication, risks, and theoretical benefits. For most people navigating primary care, this book is essential reading to be prepared for intelligent conversations with doctors and nurses when vaccines come up."

—Peter A. McCullough, MD, MPH, author of *The Courage to Face COVID-19* and *Vaccines*

"As one of Dr. Jeff Barke's grateful patients, I can personally attest to his rare combination of medical expertise and personal integrity. During the COVID-19 scare, he was my trusted go-to doctor—steady, clear-headed, and always willing to listen. He provided not just excellent care for me and my family, but reassurance and truth when it was hard to find. In this book, Dr. Barke brings that same principled approach to a complex and timely issue. His commitment to informed consent and patient empowerment reflects the kind of doctor—and man—he is. I trust him with my health, and I trust his voice in this important national conversation."

—Kirk Cameron, actor, author, evangelist, television host, documentarian, and producer

"This book is not an anti-vaccine treatise. Rather, it is cautionary work to encourage the reader to reconsider what he has been told about adult vaccines, to not blindly accept the narrative peddled by the media and the pharmaceutical industry. It is a tool to empower you, the patient, to make full use of your informed consent, to protect yourself and make the correct medical decision. As I am fond of saying, think for yourself, or others will think for you. And they will not be thinking of you. Use this book to achieve that goal."

—Mark McDonald, MD, author of *United States of Fear*

"Drs. Geehr and Barke's newest book is a vital resource for adults and caregivers seeking clarity on vaccines. It delivers well-researched insights into vaccine risks, presented in an easy-to-understand format. The book empowers readers to make truly informed choices by equipping them with tools to resist pressure from doctors pushing annual vaccinations. A must-have for anyone wanting to confidently navigate vaccine decisions with knowledge and conviction."

—Dr. Shannon Kroner, author of *Let's Be Critical Thinkers* and *I'm Unvaccinated and That's OK!*

"Drs. Jeff Barke and Edward Geehr have done an amazing book here, full of all the factual knowledge you need with his easy-to-understand delivery. It may not be politically correct, but it is well researched and from the heart, and I will recommend this book to everyone."

—Will Witt, cultural commentator and bestselling author

"*Unavoidably Unsafe for Adults* is a must-read for anyone serious about informed consent and medical freedom. Drs. Geehr and Barke pull back the curtain on the pharmaceutical agenda and expose the hidden risks of routine adult vaccinations. As a board-certified cardiologist who champions natural health, I applaud this powerful, well-researched challenge to the status quo. This book will empower you to take control of your health without blind trust in the system."

—Dr. Jack Wolfson, the natural cardiologist, America's #1 natural heart doctor

Unavoidably Unsafe for Adults

Unavoidably Unsafe for Adults

A PHYSICIAN'S GUIDE TO VACCINE SAFETY, EFFECTIVENESS, AND YOUR RIGHT TO CHOOSE

Edward Geehr, MD
and
Jeffrey Barke, MD

Skyhorse Publishing

Skyhorse Publishing books may be purchased in bulk at special discounts for sales promotion, corporate gifts, fund-raising, or educational purposes. Special editions can also be created to specifications. For details, contact the Special Sales Department, Skyhorse Publishing, 307 West 36th Street, 11th Floor, New York, NY 10018 or info@skyhorsepublishing.com.

Skyhorse® and Skyhorse Publishing® are registered trademarks of Skyhorse Publishing, Inc.®, a Delaware corporation.

Visit our website at www.skyhorsepublishing.com.

Please follow our publisher Tony Lyons on Instagram @tonylyonsisuncertain.

10 9 8 7 6 5 4 3 2 1

Library of Congress Control Number: 2025944792

Cover design by Brian Peterson

Print ISBN: 978-1-5107-8578-6
Ebook ISBN: 978-1-5107-8579-3

Printed in the United States of America

Disclaimer: This book does not offer medical advice and should be considered for educational purposes only. The information contained herein has not been approved by the FDA and should not be used for diagnosis, treatment, or prevention of any health condition or disease. The content of this book challenges conventional wisdom regarding vaccines. Consequently, it takes courage and patience on the part of the reader to consider and understand the arguments presented. Significant effort has been made to provide supporting documentation and citations. All scientific articles are subject to interpretation and the views expressed in the book may contradict the opinions of those authors and statements by the FDA, CDC, and NIH. Such is the scientific method. Please consult your health-care provider before acting on or recommending any information that may be contained in this book.

This book is dedicated to my darling wife, JT, who encouraged me to turn my frustration over the abuses and excesses of the COVID-19 pandemic into constructive action. Her editorial assistance contributed to making this book clear and accessible to the general public. I also acknowledge my co-author Dr. Jeffrey Barke and other medical colleagues who have spoken out to protect their patients against medical tyranny while at risk of losing their licenses and livelihoods. Their courage has been an inspiration and I hope this book aids in the continuing battle for medical freedom.

—Edward Geehr, MD

To all those who awakened during the tyranny of COVID—The doctors who spoke truth, the parents who protected their children, and the brave souls who refused to trade liberty for the illusion of safety.

This book is dedicated to your courage, your discernment, and your unwavering pursuit of truth and health sovereignty. May it serve as a tool in your ongoing journey of education, self-awareness, and the reclaiming of responsibility over your body and your choices.

Above all, may it point you back to the ultimate source of wisdom, healing, and freedom—our Creator, in whom true liberty is found.

"For the Spirit God gave us does not make us timid, but gives us power, love and self-discipline."

—2 Timothy 1:7

"Rebellion to tyrants is obedience to God."

—Thomas Jefferson

A special thank you to my co-author, Edward Geehr, MD—for your brilliance, integrity, and unwavering commitment to truth. Thank you for allowing me the privilege of participating in such an important and timely work.

—Jeffrey Barke, MD

Contents

Foreword

Knowledge without wisdom is simply folly. We live in "the information age," however, to many it has become difficult to filter through all the noise to come to decisions about what is verifiable and what is, shall I say, less than reliable. So how do we make personal decisions that are in our best interest? Do we defer to authority? If so, is that authority fully informed?

This book comes at a timely point in history, with new faces in positions of power in national health agencies and the clamoring of a pharmaceutically funded media in a battle over what "John and Jane Q Public" should have the right to hear. This book clearly lays out facts, history, and conflicts of interest that the lay reader, and unfortunately the majority of the medical profession, are not aware of concerning adult vaccines. Our societal conversations around childhood vaccines have evolved to a more honest discussion of their necessity, but what about immunizations for those of us that are more chronologically advanced? How do adult vaccines play into the health of adults, or do they? After reading this book, one can no longer be a medically comfortable ostrich, either as a patient or a health-care practitioner. You will be informed.

Dr. Geehr and Dr. Barke are unique in the medical world, having seventy-five-plus years of combined hands-on, face-to-face medical experience as trusted physicians, beloved by their patients and admired by their colleagues. They share a quality that many medical professionals have lost. They have maintained curiosity while much of the surrounding profession appears either willfully naive or seemingly intellectually anesthetized, overwhelmed by administrative burden and reliant on whatever the pharmaceutical reps and captured medical journal headlines tell them.

I have had the honor and privilege of getting to know Dr. Barke over the last several years during the "COVID era," first meeting him at the Defeat the Mandates rally in Los Angeles, California. Though this was a time period of exceeding frustration and division for many, in this window of world history, the silver lining was the people who were brought together in wonderfully unexpected ways. One of the bright lights for me has been Dr. Barke and his friendship of calm strength, consistent voice, and ceaseless curiosity. Having been a repeat guest on his podcast "Informed Dissent," and sharing the stage with him at several medical education seminars, I have observed his genuine care for humanity, his patients, and his colleagues and his desire to be a voice of common sense and clarity and logic. These qualities of his character will be clear to the reader as you turn the pages of this critically important, lifesaving, and health-protecting book.

Though not yet having had the honor to meet in person with Dr. Geehr, I have humbly benefitted from his excellent, incisive writings and experienced critical thoughts. His knowledge is broad and deep, augmented by his years of experience and mastery as a communicator, clinician, and educator as a University of California, San Francisco associate professor.

I invite you to delve into this book with a mind opened toward curiosity. Issues that once appeared decisively clear turn out to be more nuanced than expected. As you proceed, you might find yourself surprised to be of a newly enlightened mindset. The facts are plainly laid before you and these pages will encourage you to not only be more informed about what you allow to be, or not to be, injected into your body, but also will make you more cognizant of what is wittingly or unwittingly injected into your mind by dubious mantras of the seductive systems that would prefer you to not question or look too deeply.

We get one go-round in this life with these amazing bodies of ours. To be fully healthy is one of life's greatest gifts. All medical interventions by nature have risks and benefits. As an adult, do you truly need one of the over 170 million annual adult vaccination doses given in America? Is that risk-reward ratio an acceptable calculus for you as an individual patient with your unique genetics, existing health history, and lifestyle? Do you have all the facts necessary to make that decision? We have a right to be fully informed by our health-care providers when given the option of vaccines. It is codified into law and medical ethics. If your provider does not have a broad understanding of the margins of benefit and potential risks of an intervention, how can you be informed? Without a thoughtful and well-educated discussion with your provider, there is the potential for, at best, an unnecessary intervention, or worse, a harmful one. As you close the last page, you will certainly have acquired a lot of new knowledge. Making your own, now informed, decisions with understanding of consent will be easier. Perhaps sharing a copy of this book with your doctor might enlighten them and tickle some new neurons to fire together as well, and the shared knowledge may bring wisdom in future vaccine decisions, allowing a true, non-coerced doctor-patient partnership, rather than a paternalistic relationship.

This unique book fills a void in an overlooked area of medicine that gets brought up in almost every clinic, every day, yet is not addressed in the manner it should be. This book changes that. It puts you, the patient, in the driver's seat of knowledge with the salient data, history, and questions to confidently take to your medical professional.

Kindle the flame of curiosity and you will find an amazing story ahead which will lead you to a better opportunity to be yourself and make your own fully informed choices. Dive in, learn, grow, and enjoy. But most of all choose health.

—Ryan N. Cole, MD
Board Certified, Anatomic and Clinical Pathology Mayo Clinic and
Columbia–trained Senior Fellow in Pathology, Independent Medical Alliance
CEO, Cole Diagnostics

Introduction

"Unfortunately, a belief in the efficacy of vaccination has been so enforced in the education of the medical practitioner that it is hardly probable that the futility of the practice will be generally acknowledged in our generation . . ." [1]

—Professor E. M. Crookshank, MRCS, Professor of Comparative Pathology and Director of the Bacteriological Laboratory, King's College, London, 1889

RFK Jr.'s appointment to lead the US Department of Health and Human Services (HHS) was fueled in part by his skepticism about the safety of childhood vaccines. Vaccine safety and possible links to autism are now part of the national conversation.

The expedient application of emergency use authorizations (EUAs) for Pfizer-BioNTech and Moderna COVID-19 vaccines raised public concern about the lack of placebo-controlled trials and insufficient long-term safety data. This sentiment is now applied to other adult vaccines such as mRNA, influenza, and RSV vaccines.[2, 3] Polling data from the Kaiser Family Foundation found that one third of adults believed the COVID-19 vaccines, "caused thousands of sudden deaths in otherwise healthy people."[4]

As clinicians, we frequently field questions from adult patients about the need for so many vaccinations. Despite the rising skepticism about the safety of vaccines, American adults over fifty still receive over 177 million vaccinations annually.[5]

Vaccine	Total Annual >50 yrs Vaccinations
Influenza	115 million shots
COVID-19	53 million shots
Shingles	4.9 million shots
Pneumococcal	3.1 million shots
RSV	1.6 million shots
Total	**~177.6 million shots**

Physicians generally view adult vaccinations as an essential public health tool, with most recognizing their obligation to promote them. A 2021–2022 US survey of 1,213 health-care providers (HCPs), including physicians, found that 78.1 percent strongly believed it was their duty to promote vaccination, and 85 percent used in-person conversations to educate patients.[6]

Rarely Taught in Medical Schools

Medical schools assert they devote considerable time to vaccine education. The Liaison Committee on Medical Education (LCME), which accredits medical schools in the US and Canada, has stated that vaccine education is included in medical school training, countering claims that it's absent. In 2019, 119 out of 131 medical schools reported that they required education on vaccines and immunizations.

Dr. Stacey Rose from Baylor College of Medicine emphasized that vaccines are "absolutely part of the overall approach to teaching rising physicians about not only how to treat diseases, but also how to prevent them."[7]

Medical students are not so sanguine about their vaccine education. A 2023 survey from a US medical school found that 79 percent of medical students reported insufficient coverage of vaccine topics in their curriculum, with 54 percent advocating for more formal or mandatory vaccine education.[8]

The reality is that the vast majority of doctors generally do not receive in-depth training about vaccine science, manufacture, or regulations. If physicians believe vaccines are an essential component of preventive medicine, they should have a strong foundation for each vaccine recommendation they make, including:

- Effect of vaccines on innate and adaptive immune systems for protection against infection and transmission
- Duration of vaccine efficacy for infection and transmission
- The distinction between natural immunity and vaccine-induced immune response
- Calculation of vaccine absolute risk reduction versus relative risk reduction and how to interpret clinical trial results for patients
- Risks of biologically active excipients, and toxicity of adjuvants, with a focus on aluminum compounds in particular
- For mRNA-based vaccines, implications of modified mRNA, self-amplifying mRNA, and lipid nanoparticle transport mechanisms on vaccine distribution, toxicity, and degradation, immune dysregulation, hypersensitivity disorders, and autoimmunity

- Vaccine Approval process as distinct from other biologics and drugs, including vaccine clinical testing requirements
- Emergency Use Authorization versus Biologics License Application (BLA) Approval process requirements and implications for vaccine safety testing and effectiveness
- Manufacturer protection provisions of the 1986 National Childhood Vaccine Injury Act
- Manufacturing processes–differentiating between traditional culture media techniques, recombinant production, and custom mRNA synthesis technologies
- How to read and interpret a vaccine package insert for patients
- The distinction between a package insert, a Vaccine Information Statement (VIS), and an EUA Fact Sheet
- Post-marketing passive and active surveillance systems
- Submission of a Vaccine Adverse Event Reporting System (VAERS) report
- Query and interpretation of the VAERS database.

Difficult for Providers to Keep Up, Pressure to Conform

Many vaccine providers, struggling to stay updated with rapidly evolving research, depend on the CDC and professional associations for guidance on vaccination protocols. Organizations like the American Academy of Pediatrics, American Academy of Family Medicine, and American College of Obstetrics and Gynecologists, often funded by government entities, promote vaccines and push for censorship of "misinformation," restricting access to diverse perspectives.[9]

Many providers work within health systems that enforce standardized vaccination schedules or face peer pressure to conform. In 1980, approximately 76 percent of US physicians were owners of private practices, while about 24 percent were employed by hospitals or other entities. By 2024, the percentage of physicians in private practice (owners) had declined to 42.2 percent.[10]

Additionally, some physicians exhibit a negative bias about vaccine risks, dismissing concerns about vaccine injuries, which may limit informed decision-making for patients seeking alternative viewpoints.

Vaccine Benefits Oversold, Risks Ignored

In our opinion, as we found with childhood vaccinations,[11] the benefits compared with risks of adult vaccines continue to be dramatically oversold. In several instances, FDA approval has been based on antibody studies, not clinical trials.

Where trials have been performed, statistical techniques vastly amplify the actual effectiveness of the vaccine at preventing disease. Some vaccines have been shown to increase the likelihood of infection.[12]

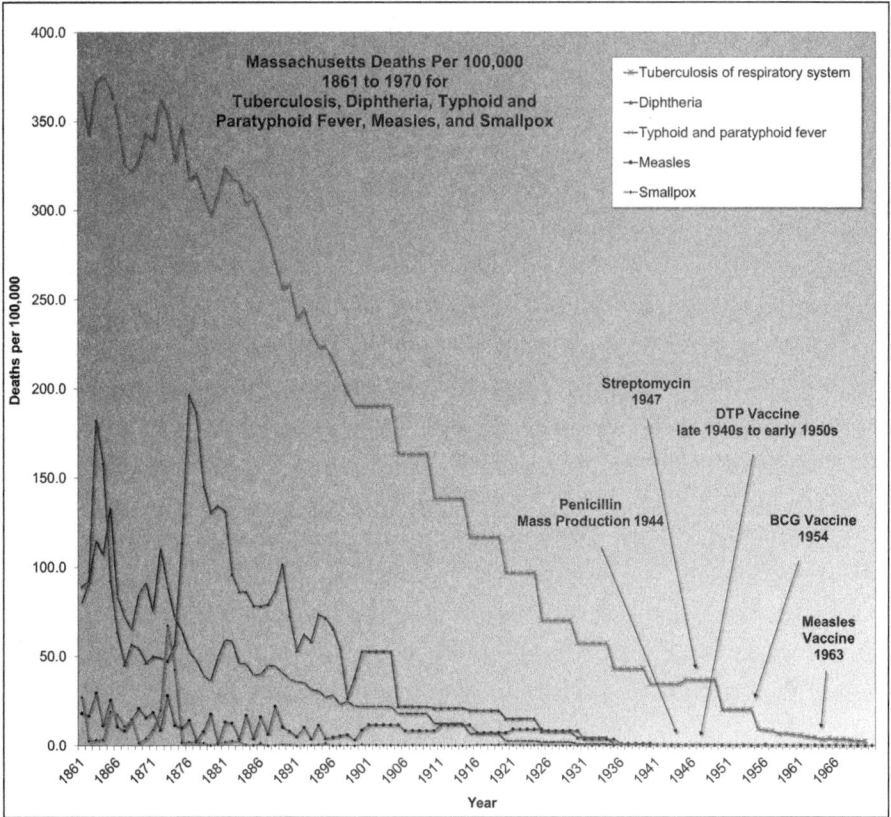

Massachusetts Deaths Per 100,000 1861 to 1970 for Tuberculosis, Diphtheria, Typhoid and Paratyphoid Fever, Measles, and Smallpox

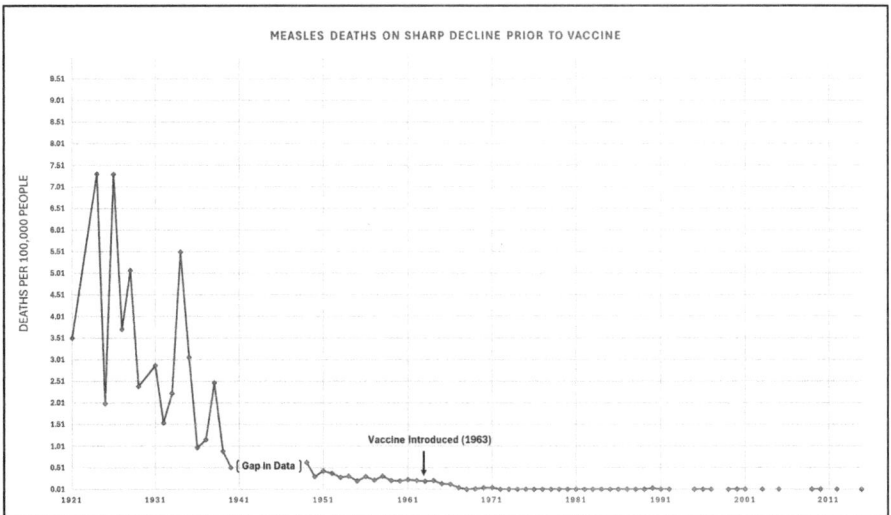

MEASLES DEATHS ON SHARP DECLINE PRIOR TO VACCINE

The history of vaccines is that they have nearly always been late to the party. Analysis of disease trends demonstrates that the incidence of deadly infectious diseases was dramatically reduced prior to the introduction of vaccines. Common fatal and debilitating infections like scarlet fever, tuberculosis, smallpox, and typhoid effectively vanished due to improvements in sanitation, water quality, and nutrition, not vaccination.[13]

Measles deaths were reduced by about 99 percent prior to introduction of the MMR vaccine in 1963.

In addition to providing actionable information to better inform decisions about vaccination, this book takes a deep dive into the evolution of legislation that protects drug makers and promotes vaccines. The role of the Department of Defense in collaboration with US Department of Health and Human Services in shaping the development of some of the most dangerous vaccines is exposed.

Nothing is off the table. The chapter on polio systematically deconstructs the mythology that surrounds the sacrosanct polio vaccine. We expose the likely sources of the twentieth-century polio epidemic and the limited role of vaccination in bringing about its end.

This book will help to inform adults and caregivers about both risks and benefits of vaccination. The pressure from personal physicians and family members to fully vaccinate each year can be relentless. The goal of this book is to promote true informed consent by providing well-sourced information in an accessible format, along with strategies for withstanding the pressure to vaccinate.

CHAPTER 1

The National Childhood Vaccine Injury Act of 1986: The Law That Opened the Vaccine Floodgates

In one of the great ironies of modern jurisprudence, the origins of the Act that indemnifies vaccine manufacturers from product liability was itself the result of defective products.
—Bruesewitz v. Wyeth LLC, 562 US 223 (2011)

In March 1979, the Government announced the recall of more than 100,000 doses of diphtheria, tetanus, and pertussis (DTP) vaccine following the deaths of four babies in Tennessee within twenty-four hours after receiving the vaccine.[1]

The CDC stated the action was being taken by Wyeth Laboratories of Philadelphia at the request of the FDA "out of an abundance of caution."[2] Wyeth, CDC, and FDA were in agreement that no direct evidence linking the deaths to the vaccine, attributing them to SIDS (a meaningless diagnosis, a catch-all acronym when the cause is unknown or inconvenient).[3]

These cases were part of a surge in lawsuits against vaccine manufacturers, particularly related to the diphtheria, pertussis, and tetanus (DPT) vaccine. During this period, public confidence in vaccines began to waver due to rare but high-profile cases of adverse reactions, notably claims that the whole-cell pertussis component of the DPT vaccine caused severe neurological injuries, such as pertussis vaccine encephalopathy (impaired brain function), childhood disabilities, and developmental delays.

Although scientific evidence linking the DPT vaccine to permanent brain injury was limited and controversial, anecdotal reports and media coverage—such as the 1982 documentary *DPT: Vaccine Roulette*—fueled public concern and sparked anti-vaccine movements.[4]

Vaccine Injuries Begin to Mount

Between 1978 and 1981, only nine liability suits were filed against vaccine manufacturers, but by the mid-1980s, this number had skyrocketed to over two hundred per year. These lawsuits often resulted in substantial jury awards, which hit pharmaceutical companies where they least liked it—their pocketbooks.

DPT vaccine was the primary focus of vaccine-related litigation during that time, largely due to concerns about the whole-cell pertussis component, which was linked to serious adverse events like encephalopathy. The MMR vaccine and oral polio vaccine (OPV) were in use at that time, but they did not attract the same level of public or legal scrutiny as DPT.

As a result, DPT manufacturers began to leave the market.

By 1985, only Wyeth (later acquired by Pfizer) was still producing the DPT vaccine, the cost of the vaccine had risen dramatically due to liability insurance costs, and availability was constrained.[5]

Generally regarded as a low-margin business, vaccine manufacturing was considered by many in the public health community to be at risk of suffering unsustainable financial losses due to vaccine injury litigation, putting further vaccine development in jeopardy.

It apparently did not occur to the public health community or vaccine manufacturers to produce a safer product. Rather, the industry with strong public health advocacy (NIH, CDC, Institute of Medicine, etc.) sought shelter from lawsuits by appealing for government protection.

Although government-industry collaborations were a common thread in these problematic mass vaccination programs (think polio), the government response was to look for a mechanism to extend even greater control over the process. After all, if a little bit of government intrusion isn't working, why not try *a lot* more?

When in Doubt, Form a Committee

In 1983, the National Institutes of Health formed The Committee on Public-Private Sector Relations in Vaccine Innovation.[6] The Committee's purpose was as follows:

> "The Committee on Public-Private Sector Relations in Vaccine Innovation was established on the premise that maintaining and extending the control of infectious diseases through immunization is an important national health objective. In compliance with its charge, it undertook a comprehensive study of vaccine research and development, production and supply, and utilization. It paid particular attention to the

institutional arrangements and interactions required to ensure vaccine availability and use, and reviewed previous efforts to identify and resolve problems in these areas."[7]

In a recommendation that was to become one of the greatest concessions to US private industry in history, the Committee advocated for a shift in vaccine liability from the manufacturers to the government (Vaccine Injury Compensation and Liability Remedies) and ultimately to the taxpayers.[8] In other words, privatize the profits and federalize the liabilities.

In addition to federal assumption of liability for all vaccine-related industry, the Committee recommended:[9]

- Supplementary (non-exclusive) compensation system
- Compensation system with restricted tort options
- Mandatory claim review by a compensation board with tort option
- Supplementary compensation system and a vaccine supply public insurance program
- Vaccine supply public insurance program and promotion of no-fault insurance for vaccine-related injury
- Changes in the tort law relating to liability for vaccine-related injury
- Acceptance of vaccine price increases to cover liability costs.

NCVIA Is Born

As a result of the Committee report, The National Childhood Vaccine Injury Act (NCVIA) was passed by Congress in 1986 to specifically exempt vaccine manufacturers from product liability based on the legal principle that vaccines are unavoidably unsafe products.

The government was now in the vaccine business as both regulator and promoter, in league with private industry. It would serve as a regulator through FDA vaccine approvals and also a partner in promoting vaccines through the CDC.

Nevertheless, the promise of vaccines as having near-mystical power to prevent disease was firmly established and broadly accepted. The NCVIA opened the vaccine development floodgates. With blanket liability protection and a favorable regulatory environment, manufacturers turned their attention to what was to become a very profitable line of business.

Number of Vaccines Explodes

Prior to 1986, there were four vaccines covering eight diseases on the market for children—Smallpox, DPT, Oral Polio Virus (OPV) and Measles, Mumps,

Rubella (MMR). Hemophilus influenza type b (Hib) was approved in 1985 but not placed on the recommended immunization schedule until 1989.

By 2010, the Childhood Immunization Schedule expanded to ten vaccines covering fourteen diseases, including DTaP, MMR, Inactivated Polio Virus (IPV), Hib, Hepatitis B, Varicella (Chickenpox), Hepatitis A, Pneumococcal, Influenza and Rotavirus.

The 2025 Schedule includes the 2010 Schedule plus Respiratory Syncytial Virus (RSV), COVID-19, and Meningococcal vaccines. By the time an American child reaches twelve months of age, they will receive twenty-eight vaccines beginning the day of their birth, and as many as ninety-two vaccines (See table below) by the age of eighteen years, the most of any country. As many as eight vaccines may be given during a single "well child" appointment.

Vaccine	Components	Doses	Total Components
Hepatitis B (HepB)	Hepatitis B	3	3
Rotavirus (RV)	Rotavirus	2–3	2–3
Diphtheria, Tetanus, Pertussis (DTaP)	Diphtheria, Tetanus, Pertussis	5	15
Haemophilus influenzae type b (Hib)	Hib	3–4	3–4
Pneumococcal (PCV15 or PCV20)	Pneumococcal	4	4
Inactivated Polio (IPV)	Polio	4	4
Influenza (Flu)	Influenza	18–20	18–20
Measles, Mumps, Rubella (MMR)	Measles, Mumps, Rubella	2	6
Varicella (Chickenpox)	Varicella	2	2
Hepatitis A (HepA)	Hepatitis A	2	2
Meningococcal (MenACWY)	Meningococcal ACWY	2	2
Tetanus, Diphtheria, Pertussis (Tdap)	Tetanus, Diphtheria, Pertussis	1	3
Human Papillomavirus (HPV)	HPV	2–3	2–3
Meningococcal B (MenB)	Meningococcal B	2–3 (optional)	2–3
COVID-19	COVID-19	10–15	10–15
Total			73–92

The Vaccine Injury Compensation Program—Going to Battle Against the Justice Department

The National Childhood Vaccine Injury Act (NCVIA) of 1986 created the Vaccine Injury Compensation Program (VICP) to compensate vaccine-related injuries while protecting manufacturers from lawsuits. However, the VICP's shortcomings undermine its effectiveness and public trust. Claimants are pitted against their own government as the program is defended by the US Department of Justice.

The program's high burden of proof for claimants, requiring stringent evidence of causation, results in only about 30 percent of claims being compensated, leaving many families without reparation. Its limited scope, confined to specific injuries in the Vaccine Injury Table, excludes complex or emerging conditions like neurological disorders, favoring arcane rules over truth-seeking.

Compensation caps, such as $250,000 for pain and suffering, often fail to cover lifelong care costs for severe injuries, exacerbating financial burdens. The VICP's opaque, lengthy adjudication process, averaging two to five years, feels adversarial despite its no-fault intent, deterring claims. Only eight thousand claims were filed from 1988 to 2020, despite millions of vaccine doses administered.

By shielding manufacturers from liability, funded by a $0.75 per-dose tax, the VICP reduces incentives for rigorous safety testing, fostering perceptions of industry bias. Critics like Robert F. Kennedy Jr. argue that this structure prioritizes vaccine supply over transparency, citing unaddressed concerns like autism. These flaws erode confidence, suggesting the VICP fails to balance safety, fairness, and accountability.

Legal Challenges—The Supreme Court's Decision in Bruesewitz v. Wyeth

It wasn't until 2011 that the scope of the NCVIA's liability protections was clarified by the US Supreme Court in Bruesewitz v. Wyeth, a pivotal case that addressed whether the Act preempts all design defect claims against vaccine manufacturers.

The case involved Hannah Bruesewitz, a child who suffered severe seizures and developmental delays after receiving a DPT vaccine manufactured by Wyeth. Her parents filed a lawsuit, alleging that the vaccine's design was defective and that Wyeth failed to develop a safer alternative.

In a 6–2 decision on February 22, 2011, the Supreme Court, led by Justice Antonin Scalia, ruled that the NCVIA preempts all design defect claims against vaccine manufacturers, regardless of whether the side effects were avoidable. The Court interpreted Section 300aa-22(b)(1) of the Act, which states that no vaccine manufacturer shall be liable for injuries caused by "unavoidable" harms if the vaccine was properly prepared and accompanied by adequate warnings.

The majority held that this provision shields manufacturers from liability for design defects, as Congress intended to create a predictable, no-fault compensation system through the NCVIA rather than allowing case-by-case litigation in state courts.

Justices Sonia Sotomayor and Ruth Bader Ginsburg dissented, arguing that the majority's interpretation overly broadened manufacturer protections and limited recourse for injured parties.

The dissenting opinion, written by Justice Sotomayor, cut to the heart of the decision. She pointed out the potential consequences of removing accountability from vaccine makers. The dissent read, in part,

> "Neither the FDA nor any other federal agency, nor state and federal juries—ensures that vaccine manufacturers adequately take account of scientific and technological advancements. This concern is especially acute with respect to vaccines that have already been released and marketed to the public. Manufacturers, *given the lack of robust competition in the vaccine market, will often have little or no incentive to improve the designs of vaccines that are already generating significant profit margins.*" (emphasis ours).[10]

Little or no incentive indeed, and the money keeps rolling into the vaccine manufacturers in record amounts.[11] But at what cost to the public?

Questionable Compliance with the NCVIA

The NCVIA authorizes the Secretary of Health and Human Services (HHS) to commission Institute of Medicine (IOM, now National Academy of Medicine) studies to evaluate vaccine safety, particularly the causal relationship between vaccines and adverse events.

HHS has commissioned several IOM studies since the NCVIA's enactment. Notable reviews occurred in 1985 (pre-NCVIA), 1991, 1994, and 2011–2013, with the latter assessing 158 vaccine-adverse event pairs, informing the Vaccine Injury Table and National Vaccine Injury Compensation Program (NVICP).

These studies addressed key safety questions, demonstrating partial compliance. However, the absence of a required frequency has led to irregular studies, with significant gaps (e.g., 1994–2011 and 2013 to the present). Critics, including advocacy groups like the National Vaccine Information Center, argue that HHS has not initiated studies proactively enough, particularly for newer vaccines or controversial adverse events.

RFK Jr. to Accelerate Vaccine Safety Studies

In 2025, newly appointed Secretary of Health and Human Services, Robert F. Kennedy Jr. outlined ambitious plans to enhance vaccine safety studies, driven by his long-standing skepticism about vaccine safety protocols. He noted that none of the mandated childhood vaccines were subjected to randomized, placebo-controlled trials.

In April 2025, an HHS spokesperson confirmed to *The Washington Post* that "all new vaccines will undergo safety testing in placebo-controlled trials prior to licensure"—a radical departure from past practices, to ensure "gold-standard science."[12]

Kennedy also prioritized investigating a potential vaccine-autism link using the Vaccine Safety Datalink (VSD), asserting that the CDC previously restricted access to this data.[13]

Kennedy's broader agenda includes improving post-market surveillance and studying alternative treatments for diseases like measles.[14] Critics, including Dr. Paul Offit, argue that placebo trials for established vaccines are unethical and could delay critical immunizations, risking outbreaks.[15] Supporters like Dr. Simone Gold praise Kennedy's push for transparency.[16]

NCVIA Should Be Withdrawn

The National Childhood Vaccine Injury Act (NCVIA) of 1986 should be repealed by Congress due to its unintended consequences on vaccine safety, accountability, and public trust. Enacted to stabilize vaccine supply by shielding manufacturers from lawsuits, the NCVIA created a no-fault compensation program for vaccine injuries. However, it has inadvertently undermined rigorous safety scrutiny and eroded confidence in immunization programs.

First, the NCVIA's liability protections for manufacturers reduce incentives to prioritize safety. By limiting legal accountability, it discourages robust pre-market testing and post-market surveillance, potentially allowing rare but serious adverse events to go understudied.[17] Critics argue that this fosters complacency, as manufacturers face minimal financial risk for harm caused by vaccines.

Second, the Vaccine Injury Compensation Program (VICP) is criticized for its high burden of proof and limited scope. Claimants must demonstrate causation within narrow criteria, leaving many with legitimate injuries uncompensated.[18] This fuels distrust among parents, who perceive the system as prioritizing industry over individuals.

Third, the NCVIA's mandate for the Institute of Medicine to review vaccine safety has not fully addressed public concerns, as evidenced by ongoing debates over autism and other conditions. The lack of placebo-controlled trials for many vaccines, as highlighted by Robert F. Kennedy Jr., exacerbates skepticism.[19]

Repealing the NCVIA would restore manufacturer accountability, encouraging safer vaccines through market-driven incentives. It would also rebuild trust by ensuring transparent, rigorous safety studies, aligning with public demand for informed choice.

CHAPTER 2

The PREP Act and Legislation That Fueled a Pandemic

"Oh what a tangled web we weave / When first we practice to deceive."
—Sir Walter Scott

How did the US government so rapidly and deceptively coordinate events during the COVID-19 crisis that were so harmful to people's lives and freedom? The answer lies in an agenda carefully and meticulously crafted over several decades.

Bioweapons for the Twenty-First Century

Following the Cold War, global superpowers like the United States and Russia no longer opposed each other with large military arsenals. US military focus shifted from a global superpower rivalry to regional "third world" conflicts and the rise of rogue states. Lacking military might, regional actors pursued asymmetrical warfare techniques with ambitions to develop weapons of mass destruction (WMDs), including biological agents.

A 1997 US Government Accountability Office (GAO) report warned that US intelligence underestimated the bioterrorism threat.[1] This report assessed the US Department of Defense's preparedness for chemical and biological defense, highlighting gaps in addressing the growing threat of biological and chemical weapons.

DOD took the report to heart and in 1998 the Pentagon drafted an internal strategy paper that promoted the development of pandemic bioweapons.[2] While cloaked as a defensive move to combat threats of bioterrorism, the document took a decidedly offensive tone.

A particularly sinister component of the Pentagon's strategy would be the ability of the military to hide the very origins of the bioweapon. The author of that paper, Colonel Dr. Robert Kadlec, wrote:

"Using biological weapons under the cover of an endemic or natural disease occurrence provides an attacker the potential for plausible denial. Biological warfare's potential to create significant economic loss and subsequent political instability, coupled with plausible denial, exceeds the possibilities of any other human weapon."[3]

An Inconvenient Treaty

The 1972 Biological Weapons Convention (BWC) frustrated US defense and spy agencies' aspirations to legally conduct research and produce bioweapons. An international treaty, the BWC banned the development, production, and stockpiling of biological and toxin weapons. It was intended to promote peaceful biological research while requiring states to destroy existing stockpiles and cooperate to prevent bioterrorism threats.

Dr. Kadlec and colleagues needed a work-around, a justification for prying open the Convention's restrictions. They needed a plan.

Dark Winter

During the summer of 2001, just three months before the 9/11 attacks, the Pentagon sponsored a war game code-named Dark Winter. Held at Andrews Airforce Base in June of 2001, Dark Winter was designed and organized by a team from the Johns Hopkins Center for Health Security and Center for Strategic and International Studies (CSIS).[4]

The exercise simulated a smallpox emergency, involving journalists to mimic media pressure. Participants concluded America lacked the ability to rapidly develop necessary vaccines and explored civil and medical countermeasures. Discussions addressed patient detention, vaccination strategies, martial law, and controlling public messaging. Public health was reframed as a military concern, integrating the US Department of Health into national security.

The distinctively military term "medical countermeasures," not medical treatments or preventive care or just plain vaccines, entered the medical lexicon for the first time. Americans could no longer assume basic civil liberties, such as informed consent or the freedom to assemble and travel, would be guaranteed. The military now had their plan for the implementation of civil and medical countermeasures, but how to pull the trigger?

Then came the 9/11 attacks. The political landscape was about to change dramatically. Safety concerns were about to supersede individual liberty.

With remarkable prescience, just seven days after the attacks on 9/11/2001 letters containing anthrax spores were mailed to several news media offices and to Senators Daschle and Leahy, killing five people and infecting seventeen others.[5]

As if excerpted from the Dark Winter script, a headline from the NIH blared, "2001 Anthrax Attacks Revealed Need to Develop Countermeasures Against Biological Threats."[6]

Perhaps not coincidentally, Senators Daschle and Leahy were among the few who initially opposed legislation imposing severe restrictions on personal privacy protections in defense of "freedom" that would become the Patriot Act. The bioweapon threat persuaded them otherwise and they became enthusiastic supporters of the bill, which passed 98–1 in the Senate.

Initially linked to foreign terrorists like Al-Qaeda or Iraq, the 2001 anthrax attacks were later attributed by the FBI to Bruce Ivins, a United States Army Medical Research Institute of Infectious Diseases (USAMRIID) scientist who later committed suicide. Other theories were proposed, such as the involvement of Steven Hatfill, a USAMRIID scientist who was investigated but completely exonerated, and government CIA participation, never fully ruled out. The case remains controversial, with no definitive proof of the perpetrator's identity, but it is difficult not to conclude the anthrax attacks fulfilled a covert agenda consistent with the Dark Winter playbook.

The Patriot Act

The Patriot Act (Uniting and Strengthening America by Providing Appropriate Tools Required to Intercept and Obstruct Terrorism Act) was signed into law on October 26, 2001. Its primary purpose was to expand government surveillance, improve intelligence sharing, and strengthen anti-terrorism measures, including tracking financial transactions and detaining suspected terrorists.

While focused on terrorism, it set a precedent for rapid legislative responses to crises, influencing subsequent laws like the Public Health Security and Bioterrorism Preparedness and Response Act of 2002. The 2002 Act, spurred by the anthrax attacks, built on the Patriot Act's urgency by bolstering bioterrorism preparedness through vaccine development, and biosurveillance, establishing the Biomedical Advanced Research and Development Authority within the Department of Health and Human Services (BARDA—discussed below).

DARPA Funds mRNA Research

The Defense Advanced Research Projects Agency (DARPA) is an agency of the US Department of Defense (DOD) responsible for developing emerging technologies for military and national security purposes.[7] It was originally created in response to the Soviet Union's launch of Sputnik 1 in 1957. DARPA focuses on high-risk, high-reward research and development (R&D) projects like artificial intelligence, cybersecurity, biotechnology, robotics, and advanced materials.

Dark Winter would become a reality. Billions of dollars would flow into bioweapon, gain-of-function research in the ensuing years. The concept of medical countermeasures would forever become associated with bioweapon-vaccine development and would become a foundational element for PREP Act legislation.

DARPA would prove to be an ideal vehicle for DOD's development of bioweapons technology. The agency had been funding RNA and DNA vaccine research since 2011.[8] DARPA's investments in mRNA technology were part of a decade-long effort to address biological threats, spurred by events like the 2001 anthrax attacks and subsequent pandemics (e.g., Zika, Ebola).

Much of DARPA's work is classified, largely shielded from public view and with limited Congressional oversight. Triple, top-secret stuff. Few understood the scope or implications of DARPA's investigations into mRNA technology until the COVID-19 pandemic.

In October 2013, DARPA awarded Moderna a grant of up to $25 million to research and develop its messenger RNA (mRNA) therapeutics platform.[9] The focus was on creating antibody-producing drugs to protect against a wide range of known and unknown emerging infectious diseases and engineered biological threats (bioweapons). This funding helped Moderna establish its mRNA platform, which later became the foundation for its COVID-19 vaccine.

Department of Defense and Department of Health and Human Services Collaboration

During the pandemic, the Department of Defense (DoD) and the Department of Health and Human Services (HHS) collaborated to procure and develop mRNA vaccines, leveraging the Defense Production Act (DPA) and Other Transaction Authority (OTA).

Using OTA, the DoD directly contracted with Pfizer ($1.95 billion for 100 million COVID-19 mRNA doses) and Novavax, bypassing Federal Acquisition Regulation rules to accelerate vaccine production through the Medical Chemical, Biological, Radiological, and Nuclear Defense (CBRN) Consortium.

In collaboration via Operation Warp Speed, HHS's Biomedical Advanced Research and Development Authority (BARDA) funded clinical trials (e.g., $1.2 billion for Moderna's mRNA-1273), while the DoD ensured production and logistics.

DARPA and BARDA mRNA Collaboration

Moderna's mRNA vaccine development also involved other US government entities, such as the Biomedical Advanced Research and Development Authority (BARDA). BARDA, along with Anthony Fauci's NIAID, would become principal funding sources for COVID-19 vaccine development. BARDA committed up to $955 million for the development of COVID-19 vaccines, particularly mRNA-based vaccines like those from Pfizer-BioNTech and Moderna.[10, 11] Before the pandemic (1985–2019), BARDA invested $148 million in vaccine development, focusing on technologies like mRNA and lipid nanoparticles.

During the pandemic (2020–2022), BARDA's investments would surge, contributing to the $31.9 billion total US public funding for mRNA vaccines, with $29.2 billion for vaccine purchases, $2.2 billion for clinical trials, and $108 million for manufacturing and research.[12]

It is difficult to imagine anything more insidious. But there was something more that would stretch credulity. The biological weapon, funded by the Department of Defense, was not directed outward to fend off a bioterrorist attack but channeled inward on an unsuspecting public with the full-throated support of the public health establishment, academia, and the media.

For a deeper dive into the current DoD Medical Biowarfare Countermeasures Program and authorities go here: https://medicalcountermeasures.gov/.

Emergency Use Authorization (EUA)

The public and most physicians had never heard of an EUA before COVID-19. Fewer still had heard of mRNA vaccines wrapped in lipid nanoparticles. Yet, less than one year after the SARS-CoV-2 virus first appeared, completely novel vaccines were authorized and aggressively promoted under the shield of an EUA. The public rocked back on its heels. Most felt compelled to get vaccinated.

Many individuals felt compelled to comply due to concerns about job security or potential discharge from the military. The FDA failed to communicate the distinction between an approved vaccine and one authorized under EUA. The principle of informed consent was cast aside.

What is Emergency Use Authorization?

The Food and Drug Administration Safety and Innovation Act (FDASIA) of 2012 expanded FDA's authority under 21 U.S.C. § 360bbb-3 (enacted under the Project BioShield Act of 2004) to issue Emergency Use Authorizations (EUAs) for unapproved medical products including vaccines during declared public health emergencies. The Act allows the FDA to authorize such products if in the agency's opinion no adequate alternatives exist, benefits outweigh risks, and a significant public health threat is present.

However, the flexibility granted by the FDA to ignore the normal approval process will tend to compromise the agency's objectivity due to political and economic pressures, indefinite EUA durations, and potential conflicts of interest. The ongoing COVID-19 EUAs, without termination as of this publication, exemplify these challenges, eroding public trust in the FDA's impartiality. The PREP Act's (see below) liability immunity further influences these decisions, highlighting the tension between emergency response and scientific rigor.

The caveat that "no adequate alternatives exist" helps to explain why the FDA was so quick to condemn repurposed medicines that showed promise in treating early-stage COVID-19 infection, such as hydroxychloroquine and ivermectin. Many clinicians also felt that monoclonal antibodies bamlanivimab, casirivimab/imdevimab, etesevimab, and sotrovimab were withdrawn prematurely and should have remained available for COVID-19 treatment.[13, 14] The FDA claimed they were ineffective against emerging variants, a claim widely disputed.[15, 16, 17] Acknowledging their effectiveness would have precluded continued issuance of COVID-19 vaccine EUAs.

How Does EUA Compare with Full Approval, Known as a BLA License?

A Biologics License Application (BLA) grants full FDA approval for vaccines, requiring extensive clinical data, rigorous manufacturing inspections, and long-term safety testing for broad use. An Emergency Use Authorization (EUA) allows temporary use during public health emergencies with less data, expedited reviews, and basic manufacturing checks. BLA ensures comprehensive validation; EUA prioritizes speed for urgent needs, with inconsistent monitoring to balance safety and efficacy.

Comparison Table: BLA vs. EUA

Aspect	BLA (Full Approval)	EUA (Emergency Use Authorization)
Purpose	Full licensure for general use in non-emergency settings	Temporary use in public health emergencies; COVID-19 injections marketed as "EUA countermeasures"
Regulatory Process	Comprehensive review (6–12 months), VRBPAC input, adheres to FDA evidentiary standards	Expedited review (weeks–months), limited VRBPAC input; only "may be effective" criterion and "circumstances that justify" apply (21 USC 360bbb)
Clinical Data	Extensive Phase 1–3 trials, long-term safety/efficacy data across diverse populations	Interim Phase 3 data, short-term safety (e.g., 2 months); not subject to full FDA safety/efficacy standards

Aspect	BLA (Full Approval)	EUA (Emergency Use Authorization)
Manufacturing Inspection	Pre-approval cGMP inspections, fully validated processes	Basic quality checks, ongoing validation; less rigorous for emergency supply
Safety Testing	Long-term data, rare event detection, Phase 4 studies	Short-term data, real-time monitoring (e.g., VAERS); no independent Institutional Review Board (IRB) or informed consent rules apply
Efficacy Standard	Robust, statistically significant across populations	"Likely effective," often based on surrogate endpoints; minimal evidentiary standards
Labeling/ Distribution	Formal labeling, broad commercial distribution	Fact sheets, controlled distribution (e.g., government-led); marketed as EUA countermeasures
Post-Market	Ongoing Phase 4 studies, routine FDA oversight	Real-time adverse event reporting, studies for BLA; absence of enforceable consumer safeguards
Duration	Permanent (unless revoked)	Temporary, tied to emergency declaration
Liability	National Childhood Vaccine Injury Act protections	PREP Act protections; recipients informed of unapproved status; potential risks with no lawful mechanisms to rectify harm
Investigational Status	Not considered investigational; fully regulated as pharmaceutical product	Described as "investigational" in Pfizer's SEC reports but not regulated as such; cannot meet standards for investigational or fully regulated products

Gain-of-Function Research—Building a Pandemic Virus

In the early 2000s, gain-of-function (GOF) research, which enhances a pathogen's virulence or transmissibility to study its pandemic potential, quietly took root in the United States, but it wasn't until 2011 that it ignited a firestorm of scientific and ethical debate. That year, virologist Yoshihiro Kawaoka at the University of Wisconsin-Madison, funded by the National Institutes of Health

(NIH), modified the H5N1 avian influenza virus to become transmissible among ferrets, a model for human spread.

Simultaneously, Ron Fouchier in the Netherlands, also backed by NIH grants, conducted parallel experiments, raising alarms about the risks of creating highly transmissible pathogens. These studies, published in 2012 after intense scrutiny, marked a turning point, thrusting GOF research into the spotlight and prompting fears of accidental releases or bioterrorism.

By 2015, Ralph Baric at the University of North Carolina at Chapel Hill, collaborating with Shi Zhengli of China's Wuhan Institute of Virology (WIV), pushed the boundaries further. Their NIH-funded study engineered a SARS-like coronavirus that infected human cells more effectively, intensifying debates about GOF's dual-use potential—its capacity for both scientific breakthroughs and catastrophic misuse.[18]

Peter Daszak's EcoHealth Alliance, a New York–based nonprofit, played a pivotal role, channeling $3.7 million in NIH grants from 2014 to 2019 to support bat coronavirus research, with a $600,000 subgrant to the WIV. The NIH, under the National Institute of Allergy and Infectious Diseases (NIAID) led by Anthony Fauci, was the primary funder.

The growing unease over the potential for GOF to create Franken-viruses led to restrictions on its use. In October 2014, the Obama administration's White House Office of Science and Technology Policy and HHS imposed a moratorium on federal funding for GOF research involving influenza, MERS, and SARS, spurred by biosafety lapses like the CDC's anthrax exposure incident. The moratorium paused new projects, but some low-risk studies continued.

In December 2017, responding to criticism from the research community, HHS lifted the ban, introducing a revised process called the P3CO Framework to review enhanced pandemic pathogen studies case by case.[19] However, scientists like Richard Ebright correctly criticized its leniency, pointing out it still allowed risky projects, including EcoHealth's Wuhan Institute work, to persist.[20, 21]

The COVID-19 pandemic escalated scrutiny. In April 2020, the Trump administration terminated EcoHealth's NIH grant amid speculation about the WIV's role in the virus's origins, with Senator Rand Paul accusing Fauci of funding GOF in Wuhan.[22]

On May 5, 2025, President Trump, supported by HHS Secretary Robert F. Kennedy Jr. and NIH Director Jay Bhattacharya, issued an executive order banning federal funding for "dangerous" GOF research, with grantees given until June 30, 2025, to comply.[23]

"Effective immediately, NIH will…[s]uspend all other funding and other support for projects, including unfunded collaborations/projects, meeting the definition of dangerous gain-of-function research" "NIH will not be accepting requests for exceptions"[24]

Public distrust persists in light of disclosures over the role of the NIH in funding dangerous GOF research. Unfortunately, the May 2025 executive order does not prohibit privately-funding GOF in the US or elsewhere. Moreover, an executive order is only as durable as the administration that issues it. The order needs to be codified into law to keep it from being reversed under a future administration.[25]

The PREP Act

The stage was set for activating the SARS-CoV-2 pandemic and a full-scale, pre-fabricated pandemic response mechanism. Gain-of-Function research funded by DOD and HHS was outsourced to the Wuhan Institute of Virology for development of the SARS-CoV-2 pathogen. When leaked from the WIV lab, HHS had the necessary precondition to declare a Public Health Emergency. Medical Countermeasures could now be released under EUA on a largely unwitting public (there were many silenced skeptics).

The final leg of the pandemic triad was a liability shield for all involved in the production and administration of Covered Countermeasures. The existing PREP Act provided just such a shield.

The Public Readiness and Emergency Preparedness (PREP) Act was enacted in 2005 to shield "covered persons" and "covered countermeasures" in the event of a declared public health emergency. It was the necessary final step in realizing the Dark Winter plan.

The PREP Act protects drug makers from financial risk related to the manufacture, testing, development, distribution, administration, and use of medical countermeasures against bioweapons and other agents of terrorism, epidemics, and pandemics. Moreover, all persons, entities, and providers who administer medical countermeasures are similarly protected.

Vaccine manufacturers heavily lobbied congress for the legislation, which would override state vaccine safety laws in the event of an emergency declaration by the Secretary of Department of Health and Human Services (DHHS). But didn't the National Childhood Vaccine Injury Act (NCVIA) of 1986 already insulate Big Pharma from product liability?

A Bioweapons Trifecta

The PREP Act completes a bioweapon trifecta. HHS can declare a public health emergency for a virus cooked up with NIH funding, medical countermeasures labelled EUA are deployed, and the PREP Act shields all the actors that inflicted a bioweapon on an unsuspecting public.

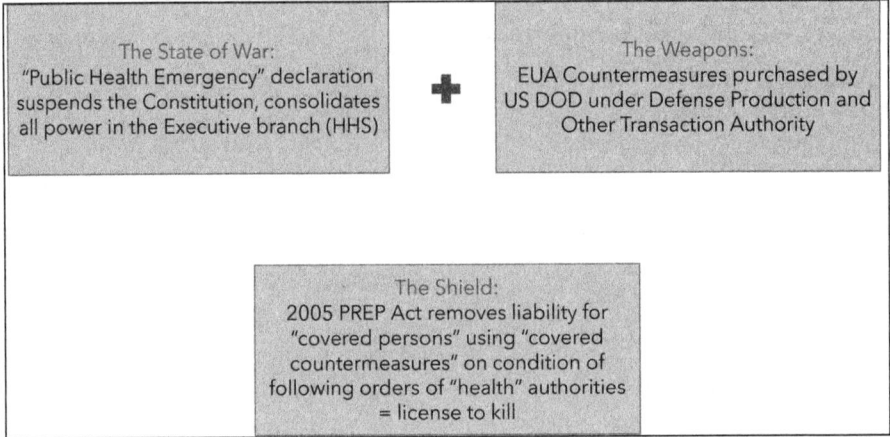

The State of War: "Public Health Emergency" declaration suspends the Constitution, consolidates all power in the Executive branch (HHS)	✚	The Weapons: EUA Countermeasures purchased by US DOD under Defense Production and Other Transaction Authority

The Shield:
2005 PREP Act removes liability for "covered persons" using "covered countermeasures" on condition of following orders of "health" authorities = license to kill

The Unholy Bioweapon Trinity[26]

Big Pharma and Big Government gained so much more than liability protection for manufacturers.

The PREP Act, combined with the Public Health Security and Bioterrorism Preparedness and Response Act of 2002, also effectively strips Americans of rights of assembly, travel, commerce, medical confidentiality, and expression of medical opinion upon the declaration of a public health emergency by the DHHS Secretary.[27]

Remarkably, just prior to the end of the Biden administration, the Public Readiness and Emergency Preparedness (PREP) Act Declaration for COVID-19 was amended on December 2, 2024, extending protections through December 31, 2029. Thus, the blanket protections for vaccine manufacturers and all other persons or entities involved in the manufacture, distribution, procurement or administration of COVID-19 vaccines continues for several more years.

As of publication, in addition to COVID-19, the PREP Act is currently invoked for countermeasures related to Marburg virus, Ebola, Zika, avian flu, RSV, monkeypox, anthrax, and smallpox. There are no pandemics or epidemics of these diseases in the United States. The declaration has no basis in reality, nor do they serve any public health interests.

PREP Act Casts a Shadow

The designation of COVID-19 as a covered countermeasure continues to exert pressure on public health policy. For example, in May 2025, HHS Director Robert F. Kennedy Jr., FDA Commissioner Martin Makary, and NIH Director Jay Bhattacharya announced:

> ". . . as of today, the covid vaccine for healthy children, and healthy pregnant women has been removed from the recommended CDC immunization schedule."[28]

Despite HHS leadership's claims, COVID-19 vaccinations are still listed on the Childhood Vaccine Schedule and Pregnancy recommendations. This listing is used to justify state and local mandates and sets a standard of care that pressures doctors and patients to comply.

Covered Countermeasures

Here are a few provisions in the PREP Act you may not have heard about.

- **Force FDA Action**

If the Secretary designates a vaccine, medication or device as a "priority countermeasure" to some perceived national threat (for example, the latest of hundreds of SARS-CoV-2 variants or monkeypox or influenza), it can direct FDA to grant fast-track approval of that countermeasure.

In fact, it can approve an unapproved drug, vaccine, device or other countermeasure based on animal experimentation alone (as has been done for mRNA boosters). No human clinical trials are required.

- **Public Surveillance Tools**

The PREP Act also directs the Secretary to evaluate new technology to improve the ability of public health officials to conduct surveillance activities related to what they perceive to be public health emergencies.

Without specifying in the Act, these could include surveillance of those who publish contrary medical opinions, who assemble for church during quarantine, who refuse a digital ID, who are unvaccinated, who use off-label repurposed drugs (think ivermectin) or even who purchases guns.

- **Detention**

Although the PREP Act does not directly grant the authority to specify communicable diseases subject to individual detention orders, a related act is often invoked in conjunction with PREP Act declarations.

Following the declaration of a Public Health emergency, a provision in the 2002 Bioterrorism Act permits the HHS Secretary in consultation with the Surgeon General to specify communicable diseases that are subject to individual detention orders.

Without specification in the Act, this could include detention of those refusing a priority countermeasure such as vaccination or isolation during a declared public health emergency. China and Australia forced detainment on thousands of their citizens and the 2002 Act provides the authority to impose the same detention on Americans.

Resentment of a Non-Compliant Public

Public health authorities at the national and local levels were highly critical and resented the unvaccinated.[29, 30, 31] They heaped scorn on those who resisted vaccination or advocated early alternative treatment with repurposed drugs in public statements, echoed by a compliant media and paid celebrity endorsers.[32, 33, 34, 35]

Do not doubt for a moment that those same authorities would readily detain citizens who openly opposed their orders if the fear factor and political will were strong enough during some future pandemic.

Who Else Has Immunity Under the PREP Act?

It's not just the vaccine manufacturers who have immunity.

For starters, you can't sue the doctor or any other licensed practitioner that injured you. The PREP Act's liability immunity applies to "covered persons" with respect to administration or use of a "covered countermeasure."

Covered persons include, "A licensed health professional or other individual who is authorized to prescribe, administer, or dispense covered countermeasures under the law of the state in which the countermeasure was prescribed, administered, or dispensed."[36]

Pursuant to such an emergency declaration, liability protection would extend to doctors and other individuals and organizations involved with countermeasures, which may include any medical product to prevent, treat, mitigate, or diagnose a potential pandemic pathogen.

So liability protection extends to the hospital that held you against your will, excluded your next of kin, forced you to take drugs you didn't want, as well as the pharmacy that gave you the injection without informed consent, the local clinic that injected or tested you, the testing laboratory that ran PCR tests with a 95 percent false positivity rate, and of course your providers.

What if you are injured from a medical countermeasure and want to sue? File a malpractice complaint in your local superior court? Not exactly. According to the Act:

> "A plaintiff whose claim is subject to PREP Act can sue the defendant only in the United States District Court for the District of Columbia. For such a civil action, PREP Act requires the complaint to be pleaded with particularity, verified under oath by the plaintiff, and accompanied by an affidavit from a non-treating physician to explain how the covered countermeasure injured the plaintiff, as well as relevant medical records."[37]

Exactly who is the defendant? The pharmaceutical company? The doctor? The clinic? No. The defendant is the United States. And who is defense counsel? None other than the US Department of Justice in a proceeding held in a special court where the normal rules of evidence do not apply.

Sue for damages due to a medical countermeasure and be prepared to surrender your rights to due process at the steps of the courthouse.

Event 201—The Ultimate Pandemic Planning Exercise

In the months leading up to the global health crisis that began in early 2020, a remarkably prescient pandemic simulation exercise known as Event 201 was conducted on October 18, 2019, in New York City.[38] It would prove to be more dress rehearsal than planning event.

Organized by the Johns Hopkins Center for Health Security in collaboration with the World Economic Forum and the Bill & Melinda Gates Foundation, the simulation modeled a hypothetical outbreak of a novel coronavirus (there are no coincidences).[39, 40] The resulting pandemic projected a catastrophic scenario with 65 million deaths.

Ostensibly, the exercise aimed to expose vulnerabilities in international health security frameworks while enhancing preparedness for real-world pandemics. The simulation underscored the complexities of coordinating global responses to pandemics, particularly when balancing scientific, economic, and geopolitical considerations.

Others claim that in reality it was a planning exercise for a pandemic that organizers knew was to come—the COVID-19 pandemic.[41] The involvement of high-profile organizations and the detailed nature of the scenario have fueled debates about the exercise's implications, particularly in light of subsequent global events. Critics have raised questions about the influence of participating entities, including the Gates Foundation and the World Economic Forum, on global health policy.[42]

Nothing can rally international cooperation, including the imposition of public health controls, like the fear of a pandemic fed by the power of the state in coordination with multibillion dollar global foundations.[43]

NIH Scientists Paid $710M by Drug Makers[44]

During the pandemic, there was a perception among some Americans that the government had close ties with pharmaceutical companies. Recently released data from the National Institutes of Health (NIH) showed that the agency and its scientists received $710 million in royalties from late 2021 through 2023.[45]

The payments are allowed under 15 US Code § 3710c to NIH researchers. NIH employees who are listed as inventors or co-inventors on patents for inventions developed at federal laboratories, or who substantially increase the technical value of such inventions, are eligible to receive royalty payments. These payments were made by private companies, such as pharmaceutical firms, to license intellectual property for medical innovations developed by government scientists. To be clear, these are government scientists on the federal payroll, working full-time, paid by the companies they are supposed to be overseeing.

Payments can be substantial, up to $150,000 per year per inventor, and can be made in perpetuity. Royalty payments continue even after an inventor leaves NIH or passes away. For deceased inventors, payments are issued to "The Estate of" the inventor.

Nor are there any disclosure requirements. Under 15 US Code § 3710c, there is no explicit statutory requirement mandating disclosure of royalty payments to NIH employees or federal laboratories. It is left to the discretion of NIH, which has been so discrete a lawsuit was necessary to crack open the books.

Most of the $710 million in royalties, $690 million, went to the National Institute of Allergy and Infectious Diseases, led by Dr. Anthony Fauci, and 260 of its scientists. Information regarding these royalties is closely guarded by the NIH. The organization OpenTheBooks.com filed a lawsuit to disclose royalties paid from September 2009 to October 2021, which totaled $325 million across 56,000 transactions. Another lawsuit was filed to obtain the new release that revealed the $710 million in payments.

Payments increased significantly during the pandemic, with more than double the cash flow to the NIH from the private sector compared to the previous twelve years combined, totaling $1.036 billion. It remains unclear whether royalties from COVID-19 vaccines produced by Pfizer and Moderna, the latter of which settled with the NIH for $400 million, are included in these figures, as the NIH has not provided further details.

In other words, vaccines are big business for government researchers as well as for drug makers. Top scientists have a powerful incentive to create novel devices, drugs, and vaccines that have great commercial potential.

Conclusion

Over the past four decades, a substantial government-industrial public health complex has evolved that poses challenges to bodily autonomy and personal liberty through vaccine development. This complex has been fashioned through numerous laws, often enacted in response to actual or perceived threats to public health.

The 1986 NCVIA laid the foundation for government-industry collaboration. The Act created a vaccine leviathan by removing product liability from manufacturers, incentivizing the addition of more and more vaccines to the Childhood Vaccination Schedule. A drug-maker backwater prior to 1986, vaccines became an irresistible cash cow for manufacturers.

Then the 9/11 attacks occurred in 2001, followed days later by the anthrax assault. This opened the bioterrorism legislative floodgates. Critical components include:

- **The Bioterrorism Act of 2002** (in response to anthrax attacks bolstered bioterrorism preparedness and established BARDA),
- **Project BioShield Act of 2004** (accelerated the development, acquisition, and availability of medical countermeasures like vaccines and therapeutics to protect the United States against chemical, biological, radiological, and nuclear (CBRN) threats),
- **DoD Medical Biowarfare Countermeasures Program** (to develop, acquire, and deploy medical such as vaccines and therapeutics to protect US military personnel from biological warfare agents),
- **PREP Act of 2005** (shields "covered persons" and "covered countermeasures" from liability in the event of a declared public health emergency),
- **Food and Drug Administration Safety and Innovation Act (FDASIA) of 2012** (expanded FDA EUA authority),
- **21 U.S. Code 360bbb-3** (further expanded FDA authority to grant EUAs), and
- **15 US Code § 3710c** (permits royalty payments to NIH researchers).

These acts in combination give the administrative state near absolute control over our lives based on a declaration by the DHHS Secretary of a public health emergency. The COVID-19 pandemic should be considered a trial run that must have succeeded beyond a government bureaucrat's wildest dreams.

Big Pharma got richer, government agencies got stronger, politicians got more power, and Americans' constitutional rights got weaker. The next pandemic will only further test the limits of their power.

Recommendations

To combat the massive growth and influence of the government-industrial public health complex, enabling legislation must be repealed or redrafted in a manner that preserves personal liberty and enables true informed consent. Action steps include:

- Withdraw the 1986 NCVIA liability protections and require enhanced safety testing of current vaccines on the Schedule
- Revise and strengthen BLA license requirement for vaccines, including randomized, placebo-controlled trials that show clinical efficacy at disease prevention and not simple immune response
- Revoke the 2005 PREP Act
- Stop all DOD—Public Health collaboration on "covered countermeasures"
- Enact legislation to stop all publicly and privately funded gain-of-function experiments
- Eliminate EUA provisions in the Food and Drug Administration Safety and Innovation Act (FDASIA) of 2012
- Revoke EUA protections in 21 U.S. Code 360bbb-3
- Restrict royalty payments under 15 US Code § 3710c
- Eliminate all vaccine mandates and require written informed consent that includes vaccine risks and benefits

CHAPTER 3

What About Polio? The Vaccine Used to Justify All the Others

"Dead flies cause the ointment of the apothecary to send forth a stinking savour."

—Ecclesiastes 10:1

"Whaddaboutpolio?" It rattles off the tongue as a single contraction, expressed more like a challenge than a question. The phrase inevitably evokes images of iron lungs, leg braces, and young lives cut short. It represents a public declaration of fealty to science and the wisdom of government regulators. Few beliefs are more sacrosanct than the life- and limb-sparing virtues of the polio vaccine.

"Whaddaboutpolio?" Anyone who challenges conventional wisdom about vaccines inevitably hears this question. The polio vaccine is the undisputed champion of public health measures used to justify all other vaccines. It's a showstopper. All conversations about vaccines begin and end with this miracle of science. Vaccine skeptics beware.

A Little History Is in Order

Poliomyelitis, or polio for short, has been around since recorded human history. An Egyptian stele circa 1500 BCE depicting a young man with a withered leg leaning on a crutch is considered the oldest representation of the disease.

Paralytic polio is rare, and fatalities are even less common. Outbreaks were rare until the late nineteenth century, interestingly restricted to developed nations. Most cases are asymptomatic, as humans tend to tolerate the virus as it passes through the intestines. Spread is caused by fecal contamination of water and food. Only a small percentage of cases, about 0.5–1 percent of infections, lead to paralytic polio.

That is what makes the outbreaks of the late 1800s and early to mid-twentieth century so unusual. They spread quickly, infecting thousands and causing high rates of paralysis and death. The search for a common source has proven elusive, although there are some compelling clues.

In the early 1900s, polio outbreaks were sporadic. A 1916 polio epidemic in New York City infected several thousand people, leading to more than two thousand deaths. Most of these were children, and death came quickly once the disease took hold. In a study of fatal cases, 82 percent died within the first week. Many of those who survived were left with lifelong disabilities.[1]

By the 1940s, polio epidemics became an annual event; over 42,000 cases were reported in 1949 alone. The early 1950s witnessed some of the worst polio epidemics in US history. The peak was in 1952, when nearly 58,000 cases were reported, resulting in 3,100 deaths and over 21,000 cases of paralysis. Families feared the summer months, often referred to as "polio season."

The Vaccine Breakthrough

The breakthrough came in 1953, when Dr. Jonas Salk announced the successful development of an injectable, inactivated polio vaccine (IPV) containing killed viruses.

"Safe, effective, and potent." That is how Dr. Thomas Francis, Director of the Poliomyelitis Vaccine Evaluation Center at the University of Michigan, described the results of polio vaccine field trials on more than 1.8 million children. Researchers estimated the Salk vaccine, produced by treating live virus with formaldehyde, to be up to 90 percent effective in preventing paralytic polio.[2]

As the nation celebrated this remarkable achievement, the government called on industry to ramp up production and disseminate the new vaccine countrywide as rapidly as possible. Several pharmaceutical companies were given licenses to make the vaccine, including Cutter Laboratories, in Berkeley, California. Cutter went all out, producing and shipping vaccine doses as fast as possible—you might even say at "warp speed."

The world breathed a sigh of relief.

Bernice Eddy, a PhD bacteriologist, worked in the Biologics Control Division of the National Institutes of Health (NIH). Her responsibilities included checking the quality of vaccines distributed by the government. In 1954, Eddy was testing different polio vaccines on monkeys when she discovered that the Salk vaccine was contaminated with live polio virus. Several test monkeys developed polio-like symptoms and paralysis. Dr. Eddy communicated her findings up the chain, but her concerns were not taken seriously. Meanwhile, the Salk vaccine and the defective mass-production method that allowed live polio virus to contaminate the vaccine proceeded without interruption.

The Cutter Incident

In what became known as the "Cutter Incident," 120,000 contaminated polio vaccine doses were released, resulting in forty thousand cases of non-paralytic polio infections, two hundred cases of paralytic polio, and ten deaths.

In May 1955, less than a month after the release of the Salk vaccine, the NIH announced that the polio mass vaccination program was shut down. Polio's highly publicized vaccine campaign became the worst public health and pharmaceutical industry disaster in history, albeit far from its last. Public pressure led to the resignations of the Secretary of Health, Education, and Welfare and the Director of the NIH.

The Sabin oral polio vaccine largely replaced the Salk vaccine in 1961.

SV40 Contamination

Simian Virus 40 (SV40) can infect various animals, including humans, and has cancer-causing potential. Dr. Eddy, who raised concerns about vaccine manufacturing in 1954, continued studying polio vaccine safety. In 1961, she found the same monkey kidney cells that served to grow the virus used in the polio vaccine could also cause tumors in lab animals.

Eddy observed, "I found something that was killing the monkeys. I couldn't just ignore it. We knew we were putting something into the vaccines that could cause cancer."[3] Despite reporting this to her pro-vaccine boss, her concerns were dismissed, and she was removed from her regulatory duties and her lab withdrawn.

Shortly thereafter, two Merck researchers identified the contaminating virus as SV40. Both the Salk (IPV) and Sabin (oral polio vaccine or OPV) vaccines had been contaminated with the virus. In 1963 the CDC (then in charge of the vaccine program) required manufacturers to switch the growth medium to another monkey species not known to host SV40.[4]

Concerns about the cancer-causing potential of the earlier versions of the vaccine were largely dismissed. Epidemiological studies on the subject were equivocal. In the 1970s, amid fears about the cancer risk of a widely administered vaccine, the CDC reassured the public about the safety of the Salk and Sabin vaccines, foreshadowing future gaslighting about vaccine safety.

Not everyone accepted CDC assurances

Dr. Michele Carbone, a researcher working for the NIH, found that SV40 could induce a rare lung cancer in animals. His work was energized by the publication in 1992 of a study in the *NEJM* that found traces of SV40 DNA in childhood brain tumors.[5] Dr. Carbone's findings were published in the journal *Oncogene* in 1994 but NIH suppressed the results and disputed any connection between contaminated vaccines and elevated cancer rates.[6]

During the ensuing years, multiple published studies found SV40 in human mesotheliomas. Drawing on available research, a book by Debbie Bookchin and Jim Schumacher challenged NIH's position. Their book, *The Virus and the Vaccine: The True Story of a Cancer-Causing Monkey Virus, Contaminated Polio Vaccine, and the Millions of Americans,* called out NIH's failure to recognize emerging evidence implicating polio vaccines as a cause of human cancers including brain, bone, kidney, lymphatics, and blood.

CDC and NIH were eventually compelled to respond. They requested the Institute of Medicine, a division of the National Academy of Sciences, convene an expert, independent panel to review the evidence. Their report, *Immunization Safety Review: SV40 Contamination of the Polio Vaccine and Cancer,* was published in 2003.[7]

The IOM imposed an unusual restriction on the committee to report only unanimous conclusions and recommendations. No majority or minority reports were allowed that might have reflected serious reservations about vaccines. Rather, the committee was constrained by unanimity. Predictably, the panel decided the evidence was inconclusive, stating: "The committee concludes that the evidence is inadequate to accept or reject a causal relationship between SV40-containing polio vaccines and cancer."[8]

The report gave the CDC and NIH cover to conclude there was nothing to see here. As far as they were concerned, except for a couple of manufacturing glitches, the polio vaccine had ushered in the modern era of safe, effective immunization, conquering the scourge of polio.

But was it really so simple? Little in health care ever is.

The common view is that polio outbreaks were public health issues resolved through vaccination, as stated by the public health agencies. However, the history of polio epidemics and their eradication involves more complex factors. Many diseases such scarlet fever, diphtheria, typhoid fever, and tuberculosis declined due to better nutrition, sanitation, and clean water.

Polio, however, occurred in areas with good sanitation and health care. A theory needs to account for these conditions and explain why polio was declining before the Salk vaccine was released in 1955.

Three often overlooked, significant factors help to explain the rise and fall of the epidemic:
- Reclassification of the diagnosis of poliomyelitis
- Environmental factors: The Great Moth Invasion
- Pesticides / DDT

Reclassification of Poliomyelitis

Definitions and accurate diagnosis matter. The diagnostic criteria for polio were refined with the advent of the Salk vaccine trials, presumably to provide more accurate tracking of vaccine efficacy. As a result, the criteria underwent reclassification to distinguish the disease from other polio-like disorders. The net result was an immediate decrease in the number of alleged polio cases in the mid-1950s, conveniently attributed to the vaccine.

Before 1954, doctors used the term polio to describe an array of diseases causing motor weakness or paralysis. These included Guillain-Barré Syndrome (GBS), transverse myelitis, acute flaccid myelitis, multiple sclerosis, spinal meningitis, Bell's palsy, botulism, Epstein-Barr virus, myasthenia gravis, peripheral neuropathy, and encephalomyelitis (brain and spinal cord inflammation) from toxic chemicals in addition to poliomyelitis.

A variety of non-polio viruses (enteroviruses EV-D68, ECHO, and Coxsackie) and autoimmune disorders can mimic the flaccid weakness and paralysis of polio.

To meet the new diagnostic criteria for polio, paralysis must be present for at least sixty days or more. This immediately precluded several other conditions. As was noted at the time, "Thus, simply by changes in diagnostic criteria, the number of paralytic cases was predetermined to decrease in 1955–1957, whether or not any vaccine was used."[9]

The practice among doctors before 1954 was to diagnose all patients who experienced even short-term paralysis with "paralytic polio." The revised diagnostic criteria required the presence of residual paralysis for at least sixty days in duration to qualify as polio. The net effect was a massive decline in paralytic polio cases.

Environmental Factors: The Great Moth Invasion

In the late 1800s, New England experienced an invasion of a non-native moth species that stripped trees bare across thousands of acres. Existing pesticides were inadequate

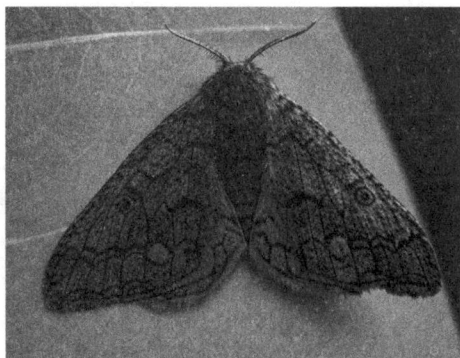

European Gypsy Moth.

for the task. Chemists tinkered with existing compounds and devised a potent combination insecticide containing arsenic and lead. Throughout 1892, lead arsenate was
applied widely throughout the greater Boston area, proving highly effective at com-
bating infestation. Little thought was given to potential human toxicity.

The following year, an unusual outbreak of twenty-six presumed polio cases
occurred in communities adjacent to the area of initial lead arsenate applications.
An atypical feature of the cases was polyneuritis. Neuritis, which is inflammation of the nerves characterized by pain, burning, tingling, and/or weakness, is
uncommon for polio. However, neuritis was a known complication of arsenic
poisoning and in retrospect the more likely cause of the outbreak.

Rutland, Vermont, 1894

In 1894, farmers in Rutland, Vermont, sought an effective insecticide due to an
impending infestation. A pharmacist provided lead arsenate, which adhered well
to produce but left pesticide residue that couldn't be washed off. Soon, over 130
cases of an "acute nervous disease," mostly in children and young adults, were
reported with symptoms unlike polio, such as high fever and seizures. Despite
Rutland's low risk for polio and clean water sources, several farm animals also
fell ill and many died. This suggested a common source of contamination other
than polio, as only higher apes and monkeys can contract it. The glaring factor in
Rutland was the introduction of lead arsenate.

New York City, 1916

In 1916, a polio epidemic struck the northeastern US, with its epicenter in New
York City. An estimated twenty-five thousand people were infected, killing around
five thousand in total. New York City bore the brunt of the outbreak, with six thousand infections and two thousand dead, mostly children. Brooklyn experienced the
most total cases although Staten Island had the greatest case load per capita.[10]

In 1916, densely populated Brooklyn was quite different than Staten Island,
which was still largely agrarian with working farms. Clearly, poor sanitation and
crowded living conditions were not the sole determinants of polio outbreaks.

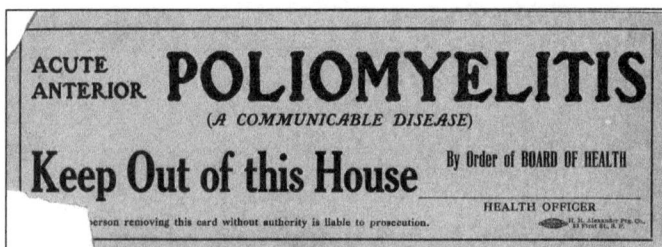

Image courtesy National Library of Medicine.

What did Brooklyn and Staten Island have in common?

At the turn of the twentieth century, production of lead arsenates migrated from local, small-batch production to larger-scale manufacturing by the chemical industry. In the early 1900s, New York City began using lead arsenate in addition to Paris Green, a highly toxic arsenical, for pest control in gardens, parks, and around homes. Farmers on Staten Island likely adopted the use of lead arsenate in addition to Paris Green to protect their crops and combat summer mosquitoes.[11]

Lab Leak Theory

Another intriguing theory about the origins of the devastating 1916 polio outbreak is its proximity to a Rockefeller Institute laboratory in Manhattan. Perhaps China's Wuhan Institute of Virology was not the first lab suspected of creating a virulent viral strain released on an unsuspecting public in 2019 (although a University of North Carolina lab may have been the original source). Over a hundred years ago, the Rockefeller lab passaged poliovirus in primate brains, meaning it repetitively cultured poliovirus to increase its pathogenicity (infectiousness and virulence).[12]

As one observer noted, " . . . it is a remarkable coincidence that a unique neurotropic strain of poliovirus was developed a few miles from an epidemic caused by a uniquely pathogenic strain of the virus."[13]

Epidemics Accelerate in the 1940s and 1950s

Periodic polio outbreaks occurred from 1916 until the 1940s, with over forty-two thousand cases in 1949. These infections cycled every few years, affecting children across all areas and classes. Researchers were puzzled by the surge and spread.

Polio typically causes minor flu-like symptoms, with paralytic cases being rare (1 in 200 to 1,000). A viral mutation might explain mid-twentieth-century epidemics, though such mutations usually reduce lethality. The unusual characteristics—summer confinement, widespread economic impact, and restriction to industrialized regions—defied contemporary explanations.

Could a modern byproduct in developed nations have caused polio's resurgence? Did late nineteenth-century outbreaks hint at future epidemics?

Pesticides / DDT

One clue might be the striking correlation between the total production of pesticides in the US, especially DDT (dichlorodiphenyltrichloroethane), and the incidence of polio. In the early- to mid-1940s, lead arsenate was still widely available as DDT production went into high gear (see first arrow on left in the illustration below). As lead arsenate production diminished, millions of pounds of DDT were produced starting in the mid-1940s, with peak production in the early 1950s (second arrow middle), foreshadowing polio's crest of nearly 58,000 cases in 1952 (see third arrow in the middle in the illustration below).

Relationship of Peak Polio Incidence and Pesticide Production

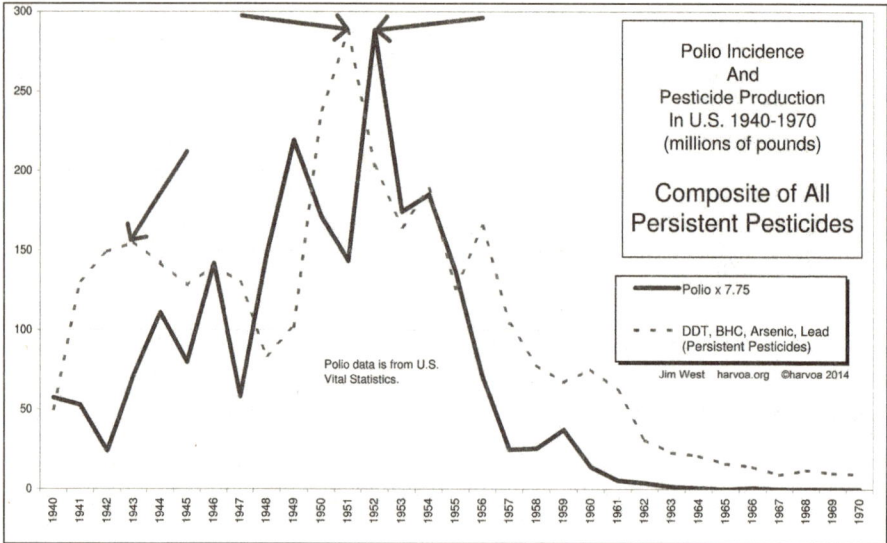

Reprinted with permission, courtesy of Jim West[14]

DDT was promoted as extremely safe and non-toxic to humans. Following World War II, it became the global insecticide of choice for households, agriculture, and public health insect-control measures.

Generous summertime spraying to control mosquitoes and other insects was the norm across the country without regard to human exposure in the late 1940s and early 1950s. Spray trucks traveled up and down congested cities and towns in the evenings, releasing vast plumes of DDT to combat the pests. The general lack of residential air conditioning ensured that windows remained wide open in summer, allowing ingress of the toxic gas.

DDT was so popular in the early fifties that it was used in children's decorative bedroom wallpaper. The product was marketed as both safe and effective against insects and came in patterns like "Jack and Jill" or "Disney Favorites." However, concern about DDT toxicity grew throughout the 1950s.

The public became fully aware of its dangers only after Rachel Carson's *Silent Spring* was published in 1962.[15] The author observed: "For the first time in the history of the world, every human being is now subjected to contact with dangerous chemicals, from the moment of conception until death. In less than two decades of their use, synthetic pesticides have been so thoroughly distributed throughout the animate and inanimate world that they occur virtually everywhere."

What Caused the Polio Epidemics of the 1940s and 1950s?

Were these cases due to polio, other infectious diseases, heavy metal poisoning, neurotoxic chemicals, or a combination? DDT exposure might suppress immunity, heightening vulnerability to viruses like polio. Polio enters through the intestines and attacks the nervous system. Children's developing intestinal immunity may be more susceptible to toxic injury than adults, reducing natural defenses against polio.

Studies show that DDT exposure can disrupt immune cell function and decrease antibody production, reducing the ability to fight infections. Combined with its toxic effects on the intestinal mucosa, this immune compromise likely played a significant role in the epidemics of the 1940s and 1950s, particularly in children.[16]

Insecticides are well-known neurotoxins and can impair cognitive and motor function. Lead arsenate has oncogenic (cancer-causing), mutagenic (genetic mutation), and teratogenic (embryonic or fetal malformation) effects in addition to neurotoxic effects. Most people afflicted with "polio" during the 1894 Rutland epidemic exhibited neurotoxic and systemic effects more typical of heavy metal and arsenic poisoning than of polio.[17, 18, 19]

The extent to which toxins or environmental factors contributed to polio epidemics in the late 1800s and twentieth century remains unknown. Pesticides might have weakened immune responses to the polio virus or other enteroviruses, leading to paralytic infections, or directly causing nervous system injury and paralysis. Early outbreaks mostly occurred in suburban and rural areas where toxic pesticides were used, suggesting a significant role for chemical agents in these epidemics.

There is little doubt that infections due to poliomyelitis caused disease, disability, and death in the US during the 1900s. Evidence for human-to-human transmission exists from various reports of public health measures including contact tracing, case-control studies, and geographic patterns of spread.[20] From the available evidence, environmental toxins likely compromised immune resistance to polio as the proximate cause of polio epidemics of the late 1800s and first half of the 1900s.

Perspective on Polio

As disabling and deadly as the polio outbreaks were in the twentieth century, it's helpful to place these epidemics in perspective. Polio did not rank in the top ten deadly diseases for the first half of the 1900s, trailing far behind TB, influenza, diphtheria, typhoid, and scarlet fever.

The 1916 polio outbreak in New York City resulted in two thousand fatalities. However, this outbreak was overshadowed by the approximately ten thousand annual deaths caused by tuberculosis in the city.[21] Despite this, polio garnered significant public attention during the 1900s primarily due to two factors.

Popular President Diagnosed with Polio
The first was the publicity surrounding Franklin D. Roosevelt's diagnosis of polio in the 1920s. As a former governor of New York who was subsequently elected President, Roosevelt was a well-known aristocrat and politician. His affliction drew attention to the disease.

A 2003 analysis speculates that Roosevelt's symptoms of fever, symmetric ascending paralysis, facial paralysis, bladder and bowel dysfunction, numbness, and hyperesthesia (extreme sensitivity to touch) were more consistent with Guillain-Barré Syndrome than polio, which typically causes asymmetric paralysis.[22] Nevertheless, the polio story took hold and helped to fuel the prevailing narrative of a national polio outbreak.

The second factor was the extraordinary success of the March of Dimes campaign launched in the 1930s by Roosevelt, where Americans were asked to send dimes to the White House to support polio research and treatment. The campaign captured the attention of millions of Americans.

Polio received significant national publicity in the 1930s and '40s, which continued into the 1950s. Other deadlier infections without as great a marketing budget declined during the same period, largely due to improved sanitation, indoor plumbing, clean water, and better nutrition. None of them had a vaccine.

Polio outbreaks were getting worse despite the national attention and financial support. The search was on for a remedy.

Turning the Tide: Polio Vaccine versus Decreased Pesticide Exposure
The introduction of the Salk polio vaccine coincided with significant changes in pesticide use. Pesticide production reached its peak around 1950, and by 1952, there were nearly fifty-eight thousand polio cases. By 1953, which was two years before the release of the Salk vaccine, polio cases had decreased to thirty-five thousand, paralleling a reduction in pesticide production.

In 1955, 6 percent (four million out of sixty-four million) of children received at least one dose of the Salk vaccine, yet polio cases dropped another 15 percent to under thirty thousand (first arrow).[23]

Polio Incidence and Declining Pesticide Production

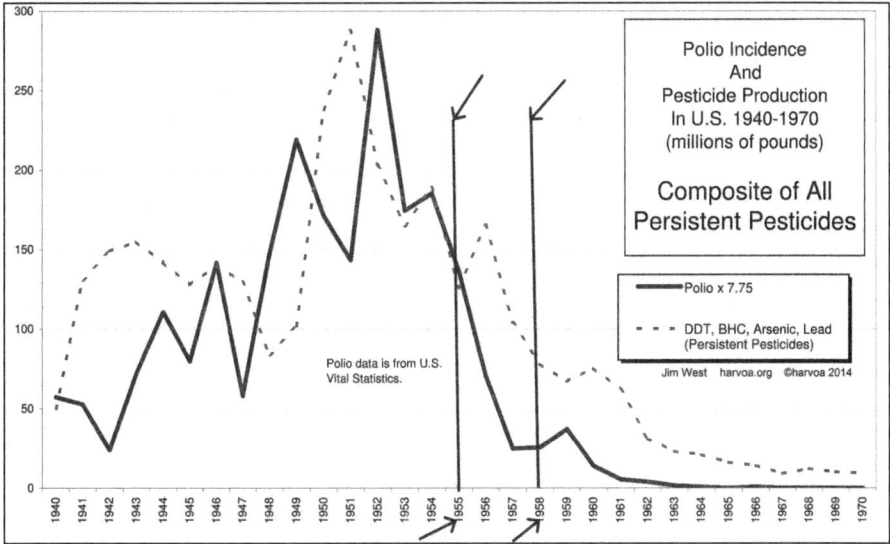

Reprinted with permission, courtesy of Jim West[24]

Three years later in 1958, approximately 40 percent of children aged ten and under remained unvaccinated, yet polio cases continued their sharp decline to just under six thousand (second arrow), a *90 percent drop from the 1952 peak.*[25]

Was it the Vaccine?

CDC attributes polio's disappearance to introducing the Salk and Sabin vaccines, without reference to declining pesticide exposure.[26]

As discussed, the decrease in pre-vaccine polio cases coincided more closely with sharp reductions in pesticide production, particularly DDT.

Likewise, it is challenging to attribute the significant decline in cases from the peak in 1952 to just three years later in 1955 solely to the release of the vaccine. Only 6 percent of American children had received one or two of the three required vaccine doses.

Crediting the 90 percent drop in cases by 1958 solely to vaccination overlooks the role of reduced pesticide production, considering only 60 percent of children under ten were vaccinated.

Failure of IPV to prevent infection or transmission

The CDC and WHO observe that inactivated polio vaccines (IPV) such as the Salk vaccine provide low intestinal immunity.[27] Therefore, individuals vaccinated with IPV can still carry and spread the polio virus. The primary effect of the vaccine is to prevent severe infection. Consequently, the vaccine is more effective in preventing serious disease than stopping the spread.

For a rapid 90 percent reduction in cases attributed to vaccination, the majority of Americans would need to have protective antibodies from vaccination or natural immunity to prevent the spread of the virus. This is known as herd immunity and represents the percentage of the population necessary to be immune before virus transmission can be blocked.

Herd Immunity

Generally, the more contagious the disease is, the greater the percentage of the population must be immune to achieve herd immunity. For example, herd immunity for the highly contagious measles virus is estimated at 95 percent while mumps herd immunity threshold is closer to 75 percent, and influenza around 60 percent.

The calculation for herd immunity depends primarily on two factors. The first is the infectiousness of the virus (referred to as the reproduction number or R0 - R zero). The second is vaccine effectiveness (expressed as a percentage).

The predominant virus of the 1940s and 1950s was Wild Poliovirus Type 1, which was highly infectious with a reproduction number estimated at six (each infected person would be expected to infect on average six others).

The Salk vaccine primarily prevented severe polio infections but failed to block infection or transmission, an important factor that led to its replacement by the Sabin oral vaccine in the early 1960s. Its effectiveness was generously estimated at 80 to 90 percent.

Based on the Wild Polio Virus Type 1 reproduction number of six and best-case estimated Salk vaccine effectiveness of 80 to 90 percent, the actual percentage of the US population necessary for herd immunity against the wild poliovirus would be over 90 percent (formula for calculation beyond the scope of this chapter but found here[28]).

Nearly achieving herd immunity by 1958 required a much higher percentage of the population to be immune to Wild Poliovirus Type 1 than were vaccinated at the time with a vaccine that still allowed viral transmission.

Assessment of vaccine effect versus environmental factors

According to the CDC, vaccines played a key role in the eradication of Wild Poliovirus in the US in the 1950s, alongside other public health measures. There is no mention of the influence of pesticides on either the onset of the polio epidemics or their decline following a significant reduction in pesticide production.

Pesticides can impact health by affecting the central nervous system and weakening the immune response to Wild Poliovirus. Considering environmental factors might provide a more comprehensive understanding of the situation. The success of polio vaccines is often highlighted as fundamental to vaccine promotion in the United States and aligns with the mission of the CDC.

The Inactivated Polio Vaccine (IPV) is frequently cited as a key example for supporting the widespread adoption and development of vaccines since the 1950s. Recognizing the contribution of other non-vaccine factors may lead to broader discussions within public health agencies and pharmaceutical companies.

The notable decline in polio cases from 1952 to 1958 was due to multiple factors, not solely the Salk vaccine. The Sabin vaccine was approved in 1961 because the Salk vaccine did not prevent polio infection or transmission but reduced the severity of the disease. The Sabin attenuated live oral polio vaccine (OPV) effectively stopped the transmission of the virus, contributing to herd immunity.

However, the Sabin vaccine also faced challenges. After its approval in 1961, there were instances of vaccine-associated paralytic poliomyelitis (VAPP) due to manufacturing quality control issues. Some individuals vaccinated with the Sabin OPV contracted paralytic polio.

Vaccines as a cause of polio—VAPP and VDPV

VAPP and VDPV Explained

Vaccine-Associated Paralytic Polio (VAPP) and Vaccine-Derived Poliomyelitis (VDPV) are lesser-known risks of oral polio vaccines (OPV). According to the CDC, VAPP occurs when the weakened poliovirus in OPV mutates, causing paralysis in the vaccinated person or close contacts. VDPV happens when this mutated virus spreads in under-immunized communities, resembling wild poliovirus. The CDC notes that OPV use in the US stopped in 2000 due to VAPP risks, though it continues in developing nations, especially in Africa, where the WHO promotes OPV for polio control despite these complications.

The media often overlooks VAPP and VDPV trends, as they challenge the dominant pro-vaccine narrative, highlighting OPV's failure to fully prevent infection and transmission.

Novel Oral Polio Vaccine (nOPV2) and Its Challenges

To address circulating vaccine-derived poliovirus type 2 (cVDPV2) outbreaks, the WHO and the Bill & Melinda Gates Foundation developed nOPV2, rolled out in March 2021. It received WHO's Emergency Use Listing in November 2020, allowing use before full safety testing. By late 2023, nearly a billion doses were administered, mainly in Africa. However, from August 2021 to July 2023, seven cVDPV2 outbreaks linked to nOPV2 were detected in six African countries, causing sixty-one paralytic cases. From January 2023 to June 2024, nineteen countries reported similar outbreaks, showing nOPV2's limited success in preventing VDPV.

Global Spread of cVDPV2

In 2022, cVDPV2 was detected in New York, joining thirty other countries, including European nations, despite high immunization rates. This suggests OPV use, not just low immunity, drives cVDPV2 outbreaks. Data from Our World in Data shows vaccine-derived polio cases now outnumber wild polio cases, posing a major public health challenge.[29]

Cases of Paralytic Polio versus Vaccine-Derived Polioviruses

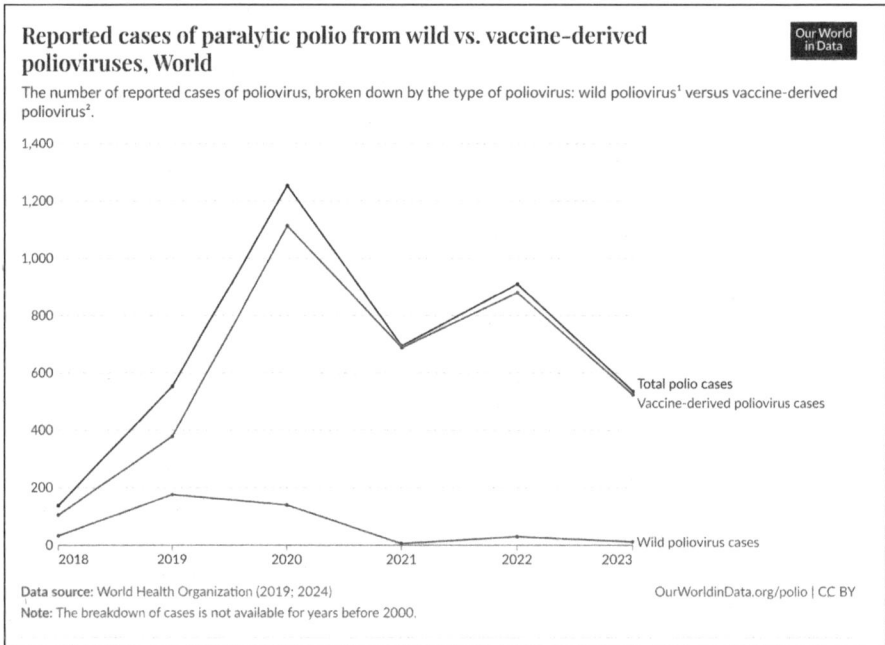

Reported cases of paralytic polio from wild vs. vaccine-derived polioviruses, World

The number of reported cases of poliovirus, broken down by the type of poliovirus: wild poliovirus[1] versus vaccine-derived poliovirus[2].

Data source: World Health Organization (2019; 2024)   OurWorldinData.org/polio | CC BY
Note: The breakdown of cases is not available for years before 2000.

Safety Concerns with IPV in the US

In the US, IPOL®, an inactivated poliovirus vaccine by Sanofi Pasteur, is used. Licensed in 1990, it was approved with only a three-day safety review and no placebo testing, despite being grown on Vero cells—monkey kidney cells prone to contamination with viruses such as measles or coronaviruses. A recent petition by ICAN demands the FDA withdraw IPOL approval pending proper safety trials, though other polio-containing vaccines remain available.

Conclusion—The Rush to Vaccinate

The lessons of polio and its vaccine development are instructive for epidemiologists, public health agencies, and vaccine manufacturers, if only they were interested. Flaws in the manufacturing process resulted in lethal contamination of the original Salk vaccine. The failure of manufacturers to follow the CDC, now FDA, guidance on Good Manufacturing Practices (GMP), and lack of FDA oversight continue to plague the industry in modern times.

The degree to which toxins or other environmental factors contributed to the polio epidemics of the late 1800s and twentieth century may never be known. Impairment of normal immune responses to the polio virus by pesticides may have resulted in the neurological injuries observed.

Regardless, the fact that the early outbreaks were primarily found in rural areas temporally related to the use of highly toxic pesticides strongly favors the role of non-infectious chemical agents as a factor in these epidemics.

CDC's disinterest in investigating all non-poliomyelitis paralysis sources likely stems from political and economic pressures that favor vaccine manufacturers. Moreover, CDC regards vaccination as core to its public health mission.[30] The pressure to vaccinate has increased over time, and a reexamination of the need and safety of vaccines is crucial for FDA/CDC to regain public trust.

Examining the origins of US polio epidemics and the public health response provides a cautionary tale. Hasty introduction of new vaccines can lead to unintended consequences and may overlook significant contributing factors.

The emergence of vaccine-derived poliovirus presents a formidable challenge to the country's public health and pharmaceutical industry alliance. A reappraisal of vaccine strategy and development, starting with proper safety testing of the approved polio vaccine, is essential to regain the public trust.

CHAPTER 4

Influenza Vaccines: Chasing an Elusive Virus

"Turning 65 was associated with a statistically and clinically significant increase in rate of seasonal influenza vaccination. However, no evidence indicated that vaccination reduced hospitalizations or mortality among elderly persons. The estimates were precise enough to rule out results from many previous studies."
—The Effect of Influenza Vaccination for the Elderly on Hospitalization and Mortality. *Ann Int Med* 2020.[1]

Influenza vaccines are a cornerstone of public health policy for protecting older adults, yet their efficacy and safety remain in question. They also represent a substantial revenue line for manufacturers Sanofi Pasteur Inc. and CSL Seqirus, generating nearly $5 billion in revenue in 2024, up over 300 percent from $1.6 billion in 2015. This chapter reviews the evidence on influenza vaccines for those sixty-five and older, addressing effectiveness, safety, and new mRNA formulations.

Influenza

Influenza is a contagious respiratory illness caused by influenza viruses that rapidly evolve new strains each year, presenting a distinct challenge for vaccine manufacturers. Flu viruses spread mainly by tiny droplets when infected people cough, sneeze, or talk. The virus can cause mild to severe illness, with the greatest disease burden falling on people sixty-five years of age and older.

Estimated Influenza Clinical Burden, Adults 65+ [2, 3, 4]

Flu Season	Illnesses (millions)	Medical Visits (millions)	Hospitalizations	Deaths
2018–2019	29 (16–46)	14 (7.7–22)	490,000 (350,000–740,000)	34,000 est
2019–2020	36 (24–50)	16 (10–22)	390,000 (300,000–550,000)	20,000 est

Flu Season	Illnesses (millions)	Medical Visits (millions)	Hospitalizations	Deaths
2020–2021	0.12 (0.068–0.22)	0.057 (0.032–0.10)	1,600 (970–3,100)	748 est
2021–2022	9.0 (5.4–16)	4.3 (2.5–7.7)	120,000 (71,000–240,000)	5,000 est
2022–2023	31 (19–47)	14 (8.4–22)	360,000 (230,000–600,000)	21,000 est
2023–2024	37 (22–65)	17 (10–49)	610,000 (610,000–1,300,000)	27,000 est
2024–2025	47 (28–110)	21 (13–60)	610,000 (370,000–1,400,000)	26,000 est (13,000–65,000 range)

Annual vaccination each fall prior to the onset of influenza season is a staple of CDC vaccine recommendations. The Center recommends that everyone six months and older get a flu vaccine every season with rare exceptions, such as allergy to a vaccine ingredient. In a June 2025 press release, the CDC reaffirmed this recommendation:

"The CDC's newly appointed Advisory Committee on Immunization Practices (ACIP) voted to recommend annual influenza vaccination for all persons aged 6 months or older with no contraindications."[5]

Vaccination is considered particularly important for people who are at higher risk of serious complications from influenza. This includes individuals aged sixty-five and older, as well as adults with one or more chronic conditions.

According to the CDC:

"People 65 years and older are at higher risk for flu-related severe illness and death. CDC research indicates that people 65 years and older account for 70 to 85 percent of flu-related deaths and 50 to 70 percent of flu-related hospitalizations each flu season. Older adults can have lower protective immune responses after flu vaccination compared to healthy young people."[6]

For adults sixty-five years and older, one of three types of flu vaccines are recommended by the CDC.

Influenza Vaccines for Adults 65 years and Older

Vaccine	Manufacturer	Vaccine Type
Fluzone High-Dose Quadrivalent*	Sanofi Pasteur, Inc.	Inactivated, high-dose, egg-based
Flublok Trivalent Recombinant	Sanofi Pasteur, Inc.	Recombinant, egg-free
Fluad Trivalent Adjuvanted**/ Quadrivalent	Seqirus	Inactivated, adjuvanted, egg-based

*Quadrivalent vaccine contains antigens from four influenza strains; Trivalent contains three strains.
**Adjuvanted indicates an ingredient added as an immune system stimulant.

RFK Jr. Cancels a Flu Shot Ad Campaign

In light of the Centers for Disease Control and Prevention's (CDC) consistent advocacy for influenza vaccination, it is noteworthy that Robert F. Kennedy Jr., the newly appointed Secretary of the US Department of Health and Human Services (HHS), decided to terminate the CDC's "Wild to Mild" flu vaccination campaign in February 2025. This campaign, initiated in 2023, utilized imagery such as a lion positioned next to a kitten to demonstrate how flu vaccines can mitigate the severity of symptoms, even if they do not always prevent infection.

According to sources, Kennedy directed the CDC to stop the campaign's paid promotions because he wanted vaccine advertisements to focus on "informed consent," emphasizing potential risks and adverse events rather than the harm-reducing benefits highlighted in the "Wild to Mild" ads.[7]

This radical shift in messaging during a severe flu season reflects Kennedy's long-standing vaccine skepticism. But was it justified? What were Kennedy's concerns?

Before considering Kennedy's rationale, here is an overview of the three influenza vaccines recommended for adults. The vaccines' ingredients, effectiveness, and risks are reviewed.

Vaccine Ingredients

Vaccines contain a range of ingredients including the virus antigen, adjuvants to stimulate an immune response, stabilizers and buffers to maintain a stable vaccine environment in the vial, preservatives to keep the antigen from degrading, and residual byproducts left over from the manufacturing process.

Vaccine	Fluzone® High-Dose	Flublok®	Fluad®
Active Ingredients	Four strains of inactivated influenza virus antigens	Four strains of recombinant* proteins	Quadravalent or Trivalent: Four or three strains of inactivated influenza virus antigens
Adjuvants**	None	None	MF59 (oil-in-water emulsion: squalene oil, polysorbate 80, sorbitan trioleate, sodium citrate, citric acid, potential autoimmune mediator, may stimulate hypersensitivity including anaphylaxis)
Stabilizers and Buffers	Sodium phosphate-buffered isotonic sodium chloride solution, Formaldehyde (potential carcinogen), Octylphenol ethoxylate detergent (Triton X-100, potential endocrine disruptor)	Sodium chloride (maintains isotonicity), Monobasic sodium phosphate, dibasic sodium phosphate, Polysorbate 20 (Tween 20, rare hypersensitivity reactions)	Sodium chloride, Potassium chloride, potassium dihydrogen phosphate, disodium phosphate dihydrate, Calcium chloride dihydrate
Preservatives	Thimerosal (multi-dose vials only): ~25 µg mercury/0.7 mL dose (potential neurotoxin)	None	None
Residual Byproducts	Egg proteins (e.g., ovalbumin, potential allergen, anaphylactic)	Baculovirus and Spodoptera frugiperda (fall armyworm) cell proteins/DNA, No egg proteins, antibiotics, formaldehyde, latex, gluten, or gelatin	Egg proteins (e.g., ovalbumin), Formaldehyde (≤100 µg/dose), Cetyltrimethylammonium bromide (CTAB), Antibiotics (kanamycin, neomycin)

*Recombinant: Recombinant DNA technology creates vaccine antigens using the virus's genetic material rather than its inactivated fragments.

**Adjuvants: Substances (e.g., aluminum salts, ethyl mercury, oil-in-water emulsion such as squalene and polysorbate 80) added to vaccines to enhance the immune response to the vaccine's active ingredients (antigens). They work by stimulating a strong immune response and by promoting inflammation at the injection site.

Vaccine Effectiveness

Fluzone® is representative of the group. It accounts for two-thirds of all adult influenza vaccinations.[8]

Influenza vaccines are updated annually based on global monitoring of strain mutations. The FDA does not require clinical trials to measure vaccine clinical effectiveness. The agency substitutes measures of antibody responses to vaccines as a proxy for clinical effectiveness.

Significantly, antibody response, also called seroconversion, does not correlate with clinical effectiveness. Therefore, an elevated antibody response to a vaccination may have no bearing on prevention of infection, hospitalization, severe illness or death.

In the case of Fluzone®, seroconversion was observed in approximately 90 percent or greater in test subjects. However, seroconversion in the control, non-influenza vaccine group was around 45 percent. This suggests that about one-half of the test subjects had natural immunity from previous flu exposures. Retrospective studies (examining data from the past) of vaccine clinical effectiveness routinely report less than 50 percent efficacy.

While no explicit VE percentage is mandated, the FDA typically expects a point estimate of efficacy of at least 50 percent against symptomatic influenza, consistent with general vaccine approval standards for preventive vaccines.[9, 10]

Fluzone® Clinical Effectiveness

Flu Season	Clinical Effectiveness for Hospitalization	Clinical Effectiveness for Infection
2020–2021	16%	Not reported
2022–2023	23%	Not reported
2024–2025	~31% (estimated, not reported)	-27%

Perhaps most troubling, annual widespread influenza vaccination has not affected influenza mortality rate of seniors which rose to estimate near-record highs during the 2024–2025 flu season.[11] (see above Summary Table of Estimated Influenza Burden, Adults 65+)

Historical Data

As with several other communicable diseases, the decline in influenza-related mortality is commonly attributed to vaccination. However, an examination of historical data on influenza mortality in the United States raises important questions about the role of the vaccine on reduction in deaths.

Rising Influenza Vaccine Coverage Has Little Effect on Mortality

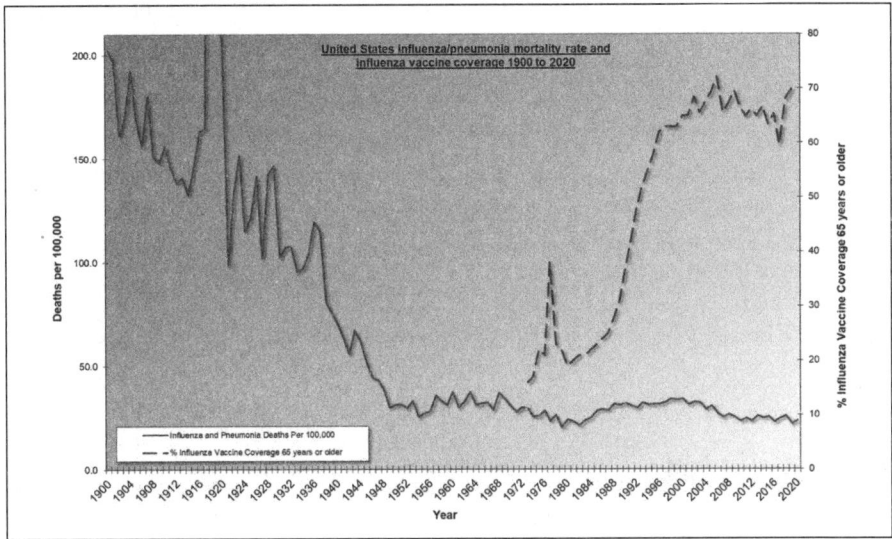

Reproduced with permission.[12]

In 1900, influenza and pneumonia caused 202.2 deaths per 100,000 people in the United States. By 1975, this rate fell to 25.8 per 100,000, an 87% decline. This achievement occurred before widespread flu vaccination, which began in the 1940s and saw routine recommendations in the 1960s. Vaccine coverage among adults aged 65 and older didn't reach 60% until the 1990s. Despite this historical decline, it remains widely unmentioned by many government and health officials.

Vaccine Safety (Fluzone® example)

Symptom	Prevalence
Myalgia (muscle aches)	18%
Headache	13%
Fatigue	13%
Malaise	10%

Common systemic symptoms post vaccination include:

Fluzone® Serious Adverse Events (SAE):

SAE	Description
Guillain-Barré Syndrome	Ascending weakness and paralysis
Encephalomyelitis	Inflammation of the brain and spinal cord

(continued . . .)

SAE	Description
Transverse Myelitis	Inflammation of the spinal cord with loss of sensory and/or motor function; loss of bowel control
Anaphylaxis	Severe allergic reaction
Facial Palsy (Bell's Palsy)	Temporary paralysis or weakness of facial muscles
Lowered Platelet Count	Reduced platelets, potentially leading to bleeding issues
Seizures	Uncontrolled electrical activity in the brain causing convulsions
Vasculitis	Inflammation of blood vessels
Cough, Wheezing, Runny Nose	Respiratory symptoms, potentially severe in allergic or hypersensitivity reactions

Revaccination Risk

A growing body of evidence indicates that repeat vaccinations year after year may not only decrease vaccine effectiveness but actually increase the likelihood of getting the flu (negative vaccine efficacy).[13]

The FLUAD® package insert indicates that in five randomized trials, repeat vaccination increased the risk of serious adverse events (6 percent of cases), including all-cause mortality (3 percent of cases), similar to another flu shot comparator. The absence of a placebo control group makes the results misleading. Just because both groups, FLUAD® versus US and non-US licensed flu vaccines, were equivalent, the finding of 6 percent SAEs and 3 percent mortality suggest a worrisome, elevated risk.[14]

A study done by the Department of Defense found repeated influenza vaccination increased the likelihood of non-flu infections up to 50 percent due to presumed immune disruption (antibody-dependent enhancement or ADE).[15] ADE or vaccine-associated enhanced disease may occur where initial immune priming (e.g., from a vaccine or infection) results in worse outcomes during subsequent infections.

Novel Vaccines in Development

Pfizer and Moderna are developing influenza vaccines based on the mRNA platform used for their COVID-19 vaccines. As discussed in Chapter 5, the mRNA platform has a dismal safety record and limited to negative efficacy on clinical outcomes. Yet, the industry persists in its pursuit of new versions of influenza vaccines using controversial mRNA technology.

Witnessing declining sales of mRNA COVID-19 vaccines, the industry hopes to leverage the popularity of annual flu vaccinations to improved acceptance of the novel technology. Moderna hopes to boost COVID-19 vaccine sales by combining the product with an influenza vaccine. Reports of the clinical trials suggest mRNA influenza vaccines remain a work in progress (see below).

Three mRNA Influenza Vaccines Currently in Phase 3 Trials:

Vaccine Name	Manufacturer	Type	Details
Moderna mRNA-1083	Moderna, Inc.	Flu/COVID Combination	Combines mRNA-1010 (flu) and mRNA-1283 (COVID-19); targets four flu strains Approval delayed to 2026 due to FDA request for more efficacy data—Withdrawn[16]
Moderna mRNA-1010	Moderna, Inc.	Seasonal Influenza (Quadrivalent)	Encodes antigens from H1N1 and H3N2 strains Ongoing efficacy study
Pfizer Quadrivalent modRNA Flu Vaccine	Pfizer Inc./ BioNTech	Seasonal Influenza (Quadrivalent)	Encodes WHO-recommended strains for Northern Hemisphere. Missed endpoints for 65+ yr olds - did not achieve the expected efficacy against laboratory-confirmed influenza-like illness

Study results thus far fail to inspire confidence. Moderna's combination vaccine has already been withdrawn one day after the FDA said it would require new clinical trials.[17] Clearly, further testing is necessary to confirm both safety and efficacy of the remaining vaccines. Moreover, mRNA influenza vaccines in particular should not obtain FDA approval until they are subjected to clinical trials against placebo controls, not solely based on seroconversion studies.

Conclusion

The effectiveness of influenza vaccines remains uncertain, and studies indicate significant potential for harms. Routine influenza vaccination in older adults has not demonstrated a reduction in hospitalization or mortality for over a decade. Secretary Kennedy likely ended the Wild to Mild campaign based on these considerations and pending further analysis by the Department of Health and Human Services (HHS). Influenza vaccines represent an extremely lucrative and reliable product line. Manufacturers will vigorously protect their cash cow from regulatory constraints. FDA should reevaluate the risks and benefits of annual flu shots for seniors and withhold approval of mRNA influenza vaccines until the safety of the mRNA platform is thoroughly assessed.

Chapter Summary

Section	Key Points
Introduction	• Influenza vaccines are considered key to public health for older adults but raise efficacy/safety concerns. • Sanofi Pasteur Inc. and CSL Seqirus earned ~$5B in 2024 from sales (up 300% from $1.6B in 2015). • Chapter reviews evidence for those 65+, including new mRNA formulations.
Influenza	• Caused by rapidly evolving influenza viruses, spreading via droplets; most severe in adults 65+. • Annual vaccination recommended by CDC for all ≥6 months, especially high-risk groups (65+, chronic conditions). • 65+ account for 70–85% of flu deaths, 50–70% of hospitalizations.
Estimated Influenza Clinical Burden, Adults 65+	• 2018–2019: 29M illnesses, 14M visits, 490K hospitalizations, 34K deaths. • 2024–2025: 47M illnesses, 21M visits, 610K hospitalizations, 26K deaths (13K–65K range). • 2020–2021 saw minimal burden (0.12M illnesses, 748 deaths) due to COVID measures.
Influenza Vaccines for Adults 65+	• Options: Fluzone High-Dose (high-dose, egg-based), Flublok (recombinant, egg-free), Fluad (adjuvanted, egg-based). • Quadrivalent (4 strains) vs. Trivalent (3 strains); adjuvants enhance immune response.
RFK, Jr. Cancels Flu Shot Ad Campaign	• In Feb 2024, HHS Secretary Robert Kennedy Jr. halted the CDC's "Wild to Mild" campaign, favoring informed consent over benefit-focused ads. • Reflects his vaccine skepticism during a severe flu season.
Vaccine Ingredients	• Fluzone: Inactivated virus, formaldehyde, thimerosal (multi-dose), egg proteins. • Flublok: Recombinant proteins, no egg/thimerosal. • Fluad: Inactivated virus, MF59 adjuvant (squalene, polysorbate 80), egg proteins. • Concerns: Neurotoxins, allergens, potential autoimmune reactions.

Section	Key Points
Vaccine Effectiveness	• Updated annually; FDA uses seroconversion (90% for Fluzone, 45% control) as proxy, not clinical trials. • Clinical effectiveness: 16–31% for hospitalization, -27% for infection (infection more likely) (2024–2025). • No reduction in mortality; 2024–2025 saw near-record deaths despite vaccination.
Vaccine Safety (Fluzone Example)	• Common: Myalgia (18%), headache (13%), fatigue (13%), malaise (10%). • Serious: Guillain-Barré, encephalomyelitis, anaphylaxis, seizures, vasculitis. • Risks linked to ingredients and immune disruption.
Revaccination Risk	• Repeat vaccination may reduce effectiveness and increase flu risk (negative efficacy). • Fluad trials show 6% serious adverse events, 3% mortality (no placebo control). • DoD study: 50% higher non-flu infection risk due to immune disruption (ADE).
Novel Vaccines in Development	• mRNA vaccines (Moderna mRNA-1083, mRNA-1010; Pfizer Quadrivalent) in Phase 3 trials. • mRNA-1083 (flu/COVID combo) withdrawn (2026 delay); Pfizer missed efficacy endpoints for 65+. • Safety/efficacy unproven; placebo trials urged over seroconversion studies.
Conclusion	• Uncertain effectiveness; no hospitalization/mortality reduction in seniors. • Kennedy's campaign halt likely based on risks vs. benefits. • Manufacturers project $5B revenue; FDA should reassess flu shots and delay mRNA approval until safety is confirmed.

CHAPTER 5

COVID-19 Vaccines: Alarming Safety Signals and Regulatory Failures

mRNA vaccines are biological timebombs. Approved by the FDA and promoted by the CDC, they comprise the most destructive force released on humans in history.

—Davis, E. Y. (May 2023). *Why you should never, ever take an mRNA vaccine*[1]

COVID-19 vaccines, especially mRNA-based formulations, play a significant role in the CDC's strategy to manage the SARS-CoV-2 respiratory virus. This chapter reviews mRNA vaccines from Pfizer and Moderna as well as non-mRNA, protein subunit vaccines from Novavax, covering their efficacy, safety, and regulatory shortcomings. The current regulatory framework for COVID-19 vaccine approvals is discussed, including the limited availability of placebo-controlled, randomized trials.

COVID-19

SARS-CoV-2, the virus causing COVID-19, spreads through respiratory droplets, leading to symptoms like fever, cough, and shortness of breath. Everyone is susceptible, but seniors (≥sixty-five years), especially those with comorbidities like obesity, diabetes or heart disease, face higher risk of severe illness. Special concerns for seniors include increased mortality rates, atypical symptoms (e.g., confusion), and long-term complications like cognitive dysfunction or organ damage.

Vaccines

What were we told when the COVID-19 vaccines were first authorized? Not only were they 95 percent effective, but that they were *safe*. The CDC assured us with specifics about Pfizer and Moderna mRNA vaccine safety.

1. The vaccines entered cells and remained *at the injection site*
2. The vaccines reprogrammed the cells to *temporarily produce the spike protein*
3. Spike proteins were neutralized by antibodies *at the injection site*
4. The mRNA would be rapidly degraded
5. Lipid nanoparticles (LNPs) used to transport the mRNA were harmless fats

Not a single one of these claims was true. It will take a generation or more for the once revered CDC to recover its reputation as a national authority on disease control.

And yet, here we are. As of the publication deadline, five total COVID-19 vaccines are approved by the FDA and promoted by the CDC from Moderna, Pfizer-BioNTech, and Novavax.

COVID-19 Vaccines

Manufacturer	Brand Name(s)	Type	Notes
Pfizer-BioNTech	Comirnaty®	mRNA 30 mcg of mRNA for ages 12 and older	Manufactured by inserting synthetic DNA plasmids into large bioreactor vats of E. coli; DNA transcribes into mRNA; purification; mRNA encapsulated in lipid nanoparticles. Purity questioned— Evidence of plasmid DNA contamination
Moderna	Spikevax®, mNEXSPIKE®	mRNA mNEXSPIKE® uses 10 mcg of mRNA compared with 50 mcg in Spikevax®	Similar process as Pfizer-BioNTech Latin word Nex means death or slaughter, often in an unusual or unnatural way
Novavax	Nuvaxovid®, Covovax®	Spike protein-based subunit	Genetically engineered in a lab using moth cells; adjuvant derived from soapbark tree extract (Matrix-M) to boost immune response.

New Regulatory Framework

With the passing of the COVID-19 pandemic, the public and many health-care providers have questioned the value of continued vaccination. Uptake of the vaccines in the most recent year was poor, according to the CDC.

Fewer than 25 percent of Americans got boosters last year, and less than 10 percent of parents vaccinated their children. Half of adults over seventy-five rejected boosters, and fewer than one-third of health-care workers joined the 2023–2024 fall booster program.[2]

In the face of this public pushback, FDA proposed a new regulatory framework for COVID-19 vaccine approval.[3] This was encouraging to vaccine skeptics as it suggested FDA would finally endorse use of the generally accepted gold standard of randomized, placebo-controlled trials prior to granting a license to market and sell the vaccine.

After all, the new Commissioner of the FDA, Dr. Marty Makary, was on record stating, "I think there's a void of data. And I think rather than allow that void to be filled with opinions, I'd like to see some good data," regarding the necessity of COVID-19 vaccines for the 2025–2026 season.[4]

Unfortunately, FDA's proposed framework fell far short of the goal to "see some good data" by accepting a much lesser standard of evidence.

First, FDA presumes that all adults sixty-five and older need to be vaccinated annually even if previously infected despite the lack of evidence for vaccine safety and effectiveness at preventing severe illness, hospitalization, or death in this group. No more studies are required for the seasoned citizens among us, no matter their health status or immunity from prior infection.

Next, the new regulatory framework deployed the expedient dodge of "immunogenicity." All that is needed to demonstrate vaccine effectiveness is to generate a certain level of antibodies in the blood. Antibody levels in response to an injection are not evidence of protection from a viral infection. This is particularly true for respiratory viruses like SARS-CoV-2 that enter through the mucosal lining of the nose and throat where other components of the immune system form the critical first line of defense.

The FDA even took it a step further away from the gold standard of evidence. They presume that antibody studies will show annual COVID-19 vaccines to be effective at preventing severe illness, hospitalization or death in children and adults with known risk factors (see CDC List below).[5] In other words, deploy first, worry about proof of effectiveness later.

The discussion below under Vaccine Effectiveness should dispel any such presumption. There is no evidence from placebo-controlled, randomized trials to substantiate COVID-19 vaccine effectiveness or safety in any age group.

For all healthy persons with no risk factors between six months and sixty-four years, FDA opened the door for manufacturers to, "conduct randomized, controlled trials in the population of healthy adults," to make their case as to why this group should also be vaccinated.[6] A hunting license, if you will, for the manufacturers to find reasons to expand the list of vaccine eligibles.

CDC 2025 List of Underlying Medical Conditions Eligible for COVID-19 Vaccination Ages 6 months to 64 years.

Condition Category	Details
Asthma	
Cancer	Hematologic malignancies
Cerebrovascular disease	
Chronic kidney disease	People receiving dialysis
Chronic lung diseases	Limited to: Bronchiectasis, COPD, interstitial lung disease, pulmonary embolism
Chronic liver diseases	Limited to: Cirrhosis, nonalcoholic fatty liver disease, alcoholic liver disease, autoimmune hepatitis
Cystic fibrosis	
Diabetes mellitus	Type 1, Type 2, gestational diabetes
Disabilities	Including Down's syndrome
Heart conditions	Such as heart failure, coronary artery disease, or cardiomyopathies
HIV	Human immunodeficiency virus
Mental health conditions	Limited to: Mood disorders (including depression), schizophrenia spectrum disorders
Neurologic conditions	Limited to: Dementia, Parkinson's disease
Obesity	BMI ≥30 or ≥95th percentile in children
Physical inactivity	
Pregnancy and recent pregnancy	Indicates presence of evidence for pregnant and nonpregnant women
Primary immunodeficiencies	
Smoking	Current and former
Solid-organ or blood stem-cell transplantation	
Tuberculosis	
Use of corticosteroids or other immunosuppressive medications	

As many as 200 million Americans meet the new regulatory framework risk criteria to be eligible for vaccination (see breakdown of estimates below). Many if not most of those eligible will be subjected to pressure from health-care providers to receive an annual booster.[7] As long as these recommendations remain in place, most practitioners will view the criteria as a standard of care, not as a basis for discussion or mutual decision-making.

COVID-19 Eligibility criteria based on age and risk factors

Eligible Population	Details
Age 65+ yr AND Age <65 yr with at least one risk factor for severe COVID-19	Estimated 33% of total US population (>100 million) will be eligible for vaccination.
Age 50–64 yr without risk factors for severe COVID-19, subjected to FDA-recommended randomized, placebo-controlled trials	Estimated 18% of total US population (61.2 million) will be eligible for FDA-designed, postmarketing trials.
Any age 6 months to 64 years without risk factors for severe COVID-19 subjected to randomized, placebo-controlled trials conducted by manufacturers.	Estimated 53% of total US population (120 million) eligible for post marketing trials conducted by manufacturers with vested interests in the outcomes.

Vaccine Schedule Based on New Regulatory Framework

To a degree, the vaccine schedule has been simplified, provided adults and their caregivers properly apply the risk criteria. The central issue discussed below is whether use of any of the approved vaccines are justified, regardless of age or health status.

2024–2025 COVID-19 Vaccine Dosing Schedule for Adults Considered At-Risk

Age Group	Vaccine Option (Brand Name)	Doses Required to Be Up to Date	Dosing Schedule
12–64 years	Spikevax® (Moderna 2024–2025 Formula)	1 dose	Single dose required if previously vaccinated or this is not the first vaccine.
	Comirnaty® (Pfizer-BioNTech 2024–2025 Formula)	1 dose	Single dose required if previously vaccinated or this is not the first vaccine.

Age Group	Vaccine Option (Brand Name)	Doses Required to Be Up to Date	Dosing Schedule
	Novavax COVID-19 Vaccine, Adjuvanted (2024–2025 Formula)	1 dose	Single dose if previously vaccinated with any COVID-19 vaccine.
	Novavax COVID-19 Vaccine, Adjuvanted (2024–2025 Formula)— First-time vaccination	2 doses	2 doses required if never vaccinated before; typically 3–8 weeks apart.
	mNEXSPIKE® (Moderna 2024–2025 Formula)— High-risk only	1 dose	Pending release. Not for primary vaccination. Expected to be available for 2025–2026 season. May be subject to further studies and earlier release for at-risk adults. Single dose for individuals with at least one CDC-defined risk factor for severe COVID-19, administered at least 2 months after the last dose of any COVID-19 vaccine.
65 years and older	Any 2024–2025 COVID-19 Vaccine (Spikevax®, Comirnaty®, Novavax COVID-19 Vaccine, Adjuvanted); (Release pending single dose mNEXSPIKE®)	2 doses	Recommended: 6 months apart - Minimum: 2 months apart (for flexibility around surges, travel, life events, or health-care visits).

Vaccine Effectiveness: Chasing an Elusive Virus

One significant challenge to developing vaccines for respiratory viruses is their rapid mutation. There are additional fundamental challenges associated with mucosal immunity that affect vaccine development for these viruses, but these are beyond the scope of this book.

Fortunately, the lethality and virulence of mutated SARS-CoV-2 strains have diminished over time. However, the mutations are difficult to predict, making vaccine composition more like educated guesswork than based on reliable predictive models. The predominant circulating SARS-CoV-2 Omicron strains have proven elusive for vaccine manufacturers. Each of the latest mRNA vaccines has failed to keep pace with the evolving Omicron strains.

According to the CDC:

"The COVID-19 vaccine helps protect you from severe illness, hospitalization, and death. It is especially important to get your 2024–2025 COVID-19 vaccine if you are ages 65 and older, are at high risk for severe COVID-19, or have never received a COVID-19 vaccine."[8]

This assertion remains unproven. The Phase III clinical trials of the BioNTech/Pfizer and Moderna mRNA COVID-19 vaccines did not establish effectiveness against severe illness, hospitalization or death despite enrolling 47,000 and 30,000 trial participants, respectively.[9, 10] The primary endpoint for both studies was prevention of infection, and as discussed below, even those claims misrepresented vaccine effectiveness.

Pfizer-BioNTech COVID-19 mRNA vaccine (2020)

- **The Pfizer-BioNTech COVID-19 mRNA vaccine** released in 2020 was tested on the Wuhan-Hu-1 strain and released under Emergency Use Authorization. This vaccine is no longer in use.
- Claim of 95 percent vaccine effectiveness against illness (not severity, hospitalization or death)
- Ninety-five percent claim is based on calculated Relative Risk Reduction or RRR
- However, the Absolute Risk Reduction or ARR calculation = 0.8 percent
- The ARR is used to calculate a more practical calculation called the Number Needed to Treat or NNT. NNT indicates the number of people that would need to be vaccinated in order for one person to avoid an infection.
- In this instance, an RRR of 0.8 percent means that the NNT = 125 (only 1 in 125 vaccinated persons will benefit from COVID-19 vaccination)
- While only 1 in 125 benefits, all 125 are subjected to the considerable number of complications and serious adverse events resulting from vaccination
- Vaccine effectiveness rapidly wanes. At best, vaccine effectiveness rapidly declined over several weeks
- Negative efficacy - Subsequent analysis by Cleveland Clinic researchers found that the greater the number of vaccinations, the greater the chances of infection. This is known as negative vaccine efficacy.[11] There are seven studies as of publication that link COVID-19 vaccination with increased risk of infection.

Studies linking COVID-19 vaccination with increased risk of infection

Study	Key Finding
Ioannou et al.[12]	Vaccinated individuals had a higher infection rate than unvaccinated controls.
Nakatani et al.[13]	Vaccinated individuals had an 85% increased odds of infection compared to unvaccinated.
Eythorsson et al.[14]	Two or more vaccine doses associated with 42% higher risk of reinfection compared to one dose or less.
Chemaitelly et al.[15]	Pfizer-BioNTech VE against symptomatic BA.1 and BA.2 Omicron infections dropped from 46.6% and 51.7% (1–3 months) to -17.8% and -12.1% (≥7 months). Moderna VE declined from 71.0% and 35.9% to -10.2% and -20.4%.
Shrestha et al.[16] (Cleveland Clinic)	Risk of COVID-19 increased with number of vaccine doses: one dose (107% higher risk), >3 doses (253% higher risk).
Feldstein et al.[17] (CDC)	Vaccinated children without prior infection were 159% more likely to get infected and 257% more likely to develop symptomatic COVID-19 compared to unvaccinated children without prior infection.
Irrgang, et al.[18]	More mRNA doses led to increased IgG4 (11x) and higher infection risk (1.8x).

Pfizer's COVID-19 mRNA vaccine (2024)

Pfizer's Comirnaty® COVID-19 mRNA vaccine for 2024–2025 targets the Omicron KP.2 strain, a subvariant of JN.1 lineage.

- FDA Approval was based on antibody studies against SARS-CoV-2 strains the company expected would be in circulation. These include KP.3.1.1, and variants that could become more common, including XEC and MC.1.

- Unlike the 2020 version of Pfizer-BioNTech's COVID-19 mRNA vaccine, the current release of Comirnaty® didn't even undergo trials for clinical effectiveness. FDA relied solely on antibody studies which poorly correlate with effectiveness at preventing infection, severe disease, hospitalization, or death.[19]

- As of this writing, the predominant strains are NB.1.8.1, LP.8.1.1, KP.3.1.1, XFG, XEC, LB.1, distant relatives of KP.3.1.1. Effectiveness against these strains is unknown and highlights the challenge of creating a vaccine to prevent a rapidly mutating respiratory virus.

Moderna COVID-19 mRNA vaccines (2020–2025)

- The original **Moderna COVID-19 mRNA vaccine** released in 2020 targeted the Wuhan-Hu-1 strain and released under Emergency Use Authorization. This vaccine is no longer in use.
  - Claim of 94 percent vaccine effectiveness against illness (not severity, hospitalization or death)
  - ARR = 1.2%
  - NNT = 83 (only 1 in 83 vaccinated persons will benefit from COVID-19 vaccination)
- **Moderna's Spikevax® mRNA vaccine** was updated in 2024 to protect against the same variant as Comirnaty®, KP.2.
  - FDA Approval was based on antibody studies against SARS-CoV-2 strains the company expected would be in circulation. These include KP.3.1.1, and variants that could become more common, including XEC and MC.1.
  - As of this writing, the predominant strains are NB.1.8.1, LP.8.1.1, KP.3.1.1, XFG, XEC, LB.1, distant relatives of KP.3.1.1. Effectiveness against these strains is unknown and highlights the challenge of creating a vaccine to prevent a rapidly mutating respiratory virus.
- **Moderna's mNEXSPIKE® mRNA vaccine** was approved for release in 2025 without a single, placebo-controlled trial despite assurances from HHS Secretary Robert Kennedy Jr. that, "all new vaccines will undergo safety testing in placebo-controlled trials prior to licensure [approval]."[20] FDA's approval failed to meet the standard advanced by Secretary Kennedy.
  - Approval based on single clinical trial conducted by the manufacturer of 11,400 participants 12 years of age and older.[21]
  - The comparator control group was Spikevax®, not a placebo.
  - The results were so poor that Moderna ignored the usually favorable RRR calculation and came up with a measure called relative vaccine efficacy (RVE).
  - RVE in preventing symptomatic Infection was reported to be 9.7 percent higher for ages 18 to 64 compared with Spikevax® and 13.5 percent higher in adults 65 and older.

Here are the clinical trial results they tried to obscure:

Group Comparison	Age	RRR	ARR
mNEXSPIKE® vs. Spikevax®	18 - 64 years	*9.32%*	1.1%
mNEXSPIKE® vs. Spikevax®	65+ years	*10.48%*	1.1%

These results do not warrant FDA approval. The agency and its advisors should be embarrassed by these results.

- **Antibody Response (Immunogenicity):** Interim results reported in a press release by Moderna from the NextCOVE trial (reported March 2024) showed that mNEXSPIKE elicited higher neutralizing antibody responses against ancestral, not currently circulating, strains Omicron BA.4/5 and original virus strains of SARS-CoV-2 compared to Spikevax.[22]

Novavax COVID-19 Adjuvanted vaccine

In 2025, the FDA approved an additional COVID-19 vaccine as outlined below. It is distinct in both its form and the nature of its clinical trial.

Novavax COVID-19 Adjuvanted 2024–2025 vaccine received FDA approval in May 2025. It is the only one of the three approved vaccines that underwent a clinical trial. The vaccine is distinctly different from the mRNA vaccines. It contains a lab-made version of the SARS-CoV-2 spike protein, which mimics the virus's molecular structure. Unlike mRNA vaccines (e.g., Pfizer's Comirnaty®, Moderna's Spikevax® or mNEXSPIKE®), which instruct cells to produce the spike protein, Novavax delivers the pre-made protein directly to the immune system.

The vaccine targets the JN.1 variant but according to the company antibody studies indicate activity against JN.1, KP.2 and KP.3 in comparison with currently circulating NB.1.8.1, LP.8.1.1, KP.3.1.1, XFG, XEC, LB.1, distant relatives of KP.3.

Novavax COVID-19, Adjuvanted vaccine:

- Only approved vaccine to undergo a placebo (saline)—controlled, clinical trial[23]
- 29,000 participants
- Vaccine =19,735; Placebo (n=9,847)
- Limited follow-up period (2–3 months)
- Claim of 90% vaccine effectiveness from 7 days after second dose (79 percent VE for 65 years and older)

- ARR = 0.84 percent
- NNT = 119 (1 in 119 vaccinated persons will avoid infection)

Assessment of COVID-19 Vaccines' Efficacy

None of the currently approved vaccines have proven efficacy against infection, severe illness, hospitalization, or death where verifiable study data is available for independent assessment. All but two of the approved COVID-19 vaccines rely on antibody response data and not disease prevention.

A recent study by Schaffer, et al. found that among healthy fifty-year-olds eligible for booster vaccination, there was no reduction in severe COVID-19 outcomes associated with the 2022 autumn booster campaign.[24] This suggests that otherwise healthy adults, including pregnant women and recently pregnant women, will obtain no benefit from COVID-19 vaccination but may incur significant risks (See Chapter 11: Vaccines and Pregnancy).

Omicron strains mutate rapidly, making vaccine predictions unreliable. The lethality and virulence of mutated SARS-CoV-2 strains have diminished over time. Each of the latest mRNA vaccines fails to keep pace with the evolving Omicron strains.

Vaccine Safety

- Comirnaty® is the most commonly used and well-studied of the COVID-19 vaccines. Commonly reported adverse reactions in adults 56 years and older.[25]
  - 38% Fatigue
  - 31% Headache
  - 18% Muscle ache
  - 14% Fever
  - 12% Joint ache
  - 12% Chills
  - 10% Diarrhea
- Comirnaty® serious adverse events[26, 27, 28, 29]
  - Myocarditis and other inflammatory conditions
  - Myocardial infarction
  - Heart failure
  - Stroke
  - Autoimmune diseases including lupus, rheumatoid arthritis and MS.
  - Blood clots and thrombosis
  - Neurological diseases
  - Multiorgan failure

- Reproductive harm
- Spontaneous abortion and still birth
- COVID-19 infection
- Immune system suppression
- Possible cancer promotion
- Out of hospital cardiac arrest
- Spikevax® commonly reported adverse reactions are similar to Comirnaty®
  - Pain at the injection site (74.8%),
  - Fatigue (54.3%),
  - Headache (47.8%),
  - Myalgia (41.6%),
  - Arthralgia (32.4%),
  - Chills (24.3%),
  - Axillary swelling or tenderness (21.7%), and
  - Nausea/vomiting (13.8%) for ages 18–64, and
  - Similar metrics for ages 65 and older
- mNEXSPIKE®
  - Moderna reports that mNEXSPIKE® was found to have a similar safety profile to Spikevax®, but both had extremely high rates of serious adverse events.
  - mNEXSPIKE® package insert reports a 2.7% serious adverse event rate compared with 2.6% for Spikevax® during 28 days of monitoring after injection.[30]
  - That means approximately 1 in every 37 people who receive either shot may suffer a life-threatening injury, hospitalization, or death in the first month alone.

Post-approval studies of mRNA vaccine adverse events

Numerous published studies following the release of mRNA vaccines have indicated that serious adverse events, those that can lead to permanent disability or death, related to vaccination continue to occur. These include declining life-expectancy, neuropsychiatric disorders, impaired immune function, stroke, heart attacks, cancer, and death. Some studies show statistical correlations, while others provide autopsy results that clearly identify widespread spike injuries as a contributing factor or cause of death.

As discussed in Chapter 6, mRNA shots can result in systemic adverse events because lipid nanoparticles (LNPs) move freely through the body, including crossing the blood-brain barrier and placenta. LNPs randomly invade tissues, making cells targets for the immune system. No organ system is safe from attack.

Listed below are several categories of serious adverse events associated with mRNA vaccines and supporting research articles.

Increased Risk of Death

Four studies highlight significant safety concerns with COVID-19 vaccines, particularly Pfizer's mRNA vaccine (see Summary of Studies table below). In King County, WA, a 1,236 percent surge in excess cardiopulmonary deaths correlated with high vaccination rates. A Florida study found Pfizer's vaccine increased all-cause mortality by 36 percent compared to Moderna's, potentially linked to 470,000 US deaths. A systematic review of 325 autopsies showed 73.9 percent of post-vaccination deaths were vaccine-related, citing multi-organ failures and inadequate preclinical testing of Pfizer's BNT162b2. Concerns include spike protein toxicity and plasmid DNA risks. A recent analysis of COVID-19 vaccination in Japan found a record number of vaccine-related deaths.

Summary of Studies on Increased Risk of Death Post-COVID-19 Vaccination

Study	Population	Key Findings
Hulscher et al. (2024)[31]	2.2 million residents, King County, WA (98% ≥1 COVID shot)	1,236% surge in excess cardiopulmonary arrest deaths (2020–2023), from 11 to 147 excess deaths, linked to vaccination rates via quadratic regression.
Levi et al. (2025)[32]	1,470,100 Florida adults (Pfizer vs. Moderna mRNA vaccines)	Pfizer mRNA vaccine increased all-cause mortality by 36%, cardiovascular by 53%, and COVID-19 deaths nearly doubled vs. Moderna; estimated 470,000 US deaths.
Hulscher et al. (2024)[33]	325 autopsies post-COVID-19 vaccination	73.9% of deaths directly or significantly vaccine-related, primarily multi-organ failures; highlights Pfizer BNT162b2 risks (e.g., spike protein, plasmid DNA, SV40) and calls for modRNA vaccine moratorium.
Kakeya H, et al. (2025)[34]	Est. 440 million doses for a population of 124 million	Japan, the most C-19 vaccinated developed country in the world at 3.6 shots per capita, records more than 1000 mRNA deaths, greater than all prior vaccines over 47 years.

Increased Risk of Adverse Events of Special Interest (AESIs)

Two studies of a combined 184 million vaccinated individuals on a global basis show COVID-19 mRNA vaccines increase risks of AESIs that could affect patient safety or public health.[35, 36] One study of 99 million vaccinated persons looked at data from the multinational Global Vaccine Data Network™ that included ten sites across eight countries. The second was a meta-analysis of fifteen studies, eleven compared the results of vaccinated with unvaccinated, and six studies compared mRNA COVID-19 Vaccines (Pfizer-BioNTech and Moderna).

Adverse Events of Special Interest (AESIs) associated with COVID-19 vaccines[37, 38]

AESIs	Increased Risk	Description
Myocarditis	+510%	Inflammation of the heart muscle, often linked to mRNA vaccines.
Heart Attacks	+286%	Myocardial infarction, increased after second mRNA vaccine dose.
Strokes	+240%	Cerebrovascular events, elevated risk after first mRNA vaccine dose.
Coronary Artery Disease	+244%	Narrowing of heart arteries, increased after second mRNA vaccine dose.
Cardiac Arrhythmia	+199%	Irregular heart rhythms, noted after first mRNA vaccine dose.
Guillain-Barré Syndrome	+149%	Autoimmune disorder causing nerve damage, linked to viral vector vaccines.
Acute Disseminated Encephalomyelitis (ADEM)	+278%	Immune system attacks myelin sheath of nerve fibers in brain/spinal cord.
Cerebral Venous Sinus Thrombosis	+223%	Blood clots in brain veins, associated with viral vector vaccines.

Possible Cancer Promotion

McKernan found plasmid DNA, including spike protein and SV40, in a colon cancer biopsy from a Pfizer-vaccinated patient, suggesting replication and potential DNA integration risks. Alden et al. found that Pfizer-BioNTech mRNA vaccine was rapidly reverse transcribed into liver cells, posing the risk of permanent genetic alteration. A review by Angueira highlights cancer's complexity, noting mRNA vaccines may worsen cancer by suppressing immunity or promoting inflammation. A study out of Turkey found distinctive metabolic profile differences between leukemia patients who were vaccinated compared with controls and unvaccinated leukemia patients. All call for further research into vaccine safety, DNA plasmid contamination, and cancer interactions.

mRNA COVID-19 Vaccines and Cancer Risks

Study/Source	Key Findings	Implications
McKernan[39] (2024)	Plasmid DNA, including spike protein and SV40, detected in colon cancer biopsy; high copy numbers suggest replication, raising DNA integration and cancer risk concerns.	Potential for vaccine-derived DNA to increase oncogenesis, though origin and causality are unclear; calls for further research.
Alden et al.[40] (2022)	Pfizer-BioNTech mRNA was reverse-transcribed into DNA within the liver cells as quickly as six hours after exposure.	The rapid reverse transcription and potential for DNA formation raise concerns about the safety of mRNA vaccines, particularly regarding the possibility of unintended genetic changes.
Angueira[41] (2024)	Cancer's complexity complicates vaccine recommendations; mRNA vaccines may suppress immunity, promote inflammation, or activate harmful processes, potentially worsening or triggering cancer in excluded trial patients.	Uncertain safety for cancer patients; vaccines might exacerbate cancer, necessitating further study despite lack of definitive evidence.
Erdoğdu et al.[42] (2024)	Leukemia diagnosed after mRNA vaccination showed distinct metabolic alterations compared with controls and unvaccinated leukemia patients.	Vaccinated leukemia patients (n=7)—all of whom developed leukemia within 15 to 63 days after receiving Pfizer's BNT162b2 COVID-19 mRNA injection
Abue et al.[43]	Repeated COVID-19 vaccinations increase spike-specific IgG4, raising concerns about cancer immunity in pancreatic cancer patients. Frequent booster shots are linked to worse overall survival in PC patients.	Repeated COVID-19 vaccinations alter levels of IgG4, interfering with cancer immunity which may decrease survival in cancer patients.

Immune Dysregulation Linked to COVID-19 Vaccination

A Yale study by Bhattacharjee and Iwasaki reveals post-vaccination syndrome (PVS) linked to mRNA COVID vaccines, characterized by symptoms like brain fog, dizziness, and fatigue.[44] Analyzing forty-two PVS and twenty-two healthy participants, researchers found T-cell exhaustion (Vaccine-Acquired Immunodeficiency Syndrome or VAIDS), persistent spike protein production (up to 709 days post-vaccination), and Epstein-Barr virus (EBV) reactivation in PVS patients. These immune dysfunctions mirror long COVID, with PVS showing higher spike protein levels.

Key Findings from Yale Study on mRNA COVID Vaccine Effects

Finding	Description	Implication
T-Cell Exhaustion (VAIDS)	Dysregulation of T cells that control immune function and inflammatory responses	Indicates vaccine-induced immune dysfunction, akin to acquired immunodeficiency
Persistent Spike Protein	Detectable spike protein up to 709 days post-vaccination, increasing over time	Drives chronic inflammation, contributing to PVS and long COVID symptoms
EBV Reactivation	Elevated anti-EBV IgG in PVS and long COVID patients	Reactivated virus may cause fatigue, nerve issues, and exacerbate symptoms

Vascular Damage from Spike Proteins

An analysis of nineteen hemorrhagic stroke cases (2023–2024) found SARS-CoV-2 spike protein in cerebral arteries of 43.8 percent of mRNA-vaccinated patients, persisting up to seventeen months post-vaccination, exclusively in females. Inflammatory cell infiltration was observed, raising concerns about lipid nanoparticle biodistribution and long-term safety.[45] The Yale study complements this, linking persistent spike protein to immune dysfunction (T-cell exhaustion, EBV reactivation) in post-vaccination syndrome. Both studies highlight mRNA vaccine safety issues, urging global replication studies to assess cerebrovascular and systemic risks.

Myocarditis and Other Inflammatory Conditions

The public is increasingly aware of and concerned about the association of COVID-19 vaccination and heart problems. A recent survey found that 51 percent of American adults believe it's likely that the COVID-19 vaccine has caused inflammation in the hearts of many vaccinated Americans, including 29 percent who think it is very likely.[46]

This follows FDA's order to COVID-19 vaccine manufacturers to expand their warnings about the risk of heart-related side effects, including myocarditis and pericarditis. Several studies have identified cardiac injury following COVID-19 vaccination.

One such study authored by Mead, et. al., published in the *International Journal of Cardiovascular Research & Innovation* in 2025, challenges public health claims about COVID-19 mRNA vaccine safety.[47] Backed by 341 references, the study synthesizes clinical trial results, post-marketing surveillance, and observational data to compare myocarditis from SARS-CoV-2 infection versus mRNA vaccination.

The study reports that vaccine-induced myocarditis is more common and severe than infection-related cases, particularly in young males under forty. Key findings include a 96 percent hospitalization rate for CDC-confirmed vaccine-related myocarditis cases, over 50 percent of cases showing long-term heart damage on MRI, and a fatality rate of up to 20 percent.

A Swiss study noted 2.8 percent subclinical heart injury post-mRNA booster, and young men face a sixfold higher myocarditis risk after the second Moderna dose compared to infection.[48] Autopsies link 7.1 percent of vaccine-related deaths to myocarditis. The study refutes claims that vaccine-induced myocarditis is mild, transient, or rarer than infection-related cases, urging immediate withdrawal of mRNA vaccines due to significant cardiotoxicity risks.

Mead Study Table of Results

Metric	Finding	Details
Hospitalization Rate	96%	96% of CDC-confirmed mRNA vaccine-induced myocarditis cases required hospitalization.
Subclinical Injury	2.8%	Swiss study found 2.8% of individuals had subclinical heart injury after mRNA booster.
Long-term Heart Damage	>50%	Over 50% of vaccine-induced myocarditis cases show lasting heart damage on cardiac MRI (e.g., late gadolinium enhancement).
Fatality Rate	10–20%	Estimated fatality rate for confirmed vaccine-induced myocarditis cases, significantly higher than reported.
Risk in Young Men	6× Higher	Young males (<40) have a sixfold higher myocarditis risk after second Moderna dose compared to SARS-CoV-2 infection.
Vaccine-Related Deaths	7.1%	Autopsy-confirmed myocarditis accounts for 7.1% of deaths attributed to mRNA vaccines.

Other studies are consistent with the McCullough Foundation Report

- A study of 40 mRNA COVID-19 vaccine recipients with myocarditis found half had mild inflammation without heart muscle damage, while half had damaged heart muscle, often with severe inflammation. Those with damage were older, had less chest pain, weaker heart function, and worse outcomes, often requiring heart support machines.[49]
- A comprehensive review analyzed the epidemiology and outcomes of myocarditis following both SARS-CoV-2 infection and COVID-19 vaccination. The study highlighted the need for continued surveillance and research into the long-term effects of such cardiac injuries.[50]
- A Korean study used cardiac imaging techniques to assess a large cohort of individuals post-SARS-CoV-2 infection and vaccination. It identified cardiac abnormalities, including myocardial inflammation and fibrosis, in a subset of vaccinated individuals, particularly after mRNA vaccines.[51]
- A peer-reviewed study has uncovered a significant increase in a deadly heart condition among those who received Covid mRNA vaccines. The analysis showed that recipients experienced adverse events at 26 times the rate of flu vaccine recipients. It also revealed that Covid mRNA injections caused myocarditis, a dangerous heart inflammation, at 1152 times higher incidence than the flu shot.[52]

Thyroid Disorders

A study involving over 2.3 million patients indicates that individuals who received mRNA COVID-19 vaccines were 30 percent more likely to develop thyroid disease within a year compared to those who did not receive the vaccine. The incidence of thyroid disease worsened progressively, with the disparity between vaccinated and unvaccinated individuals increasing steadily, according to researchers. Thyroid disease is prevalent, and the study identified over four thousand additional cases in the vaccinated cohort, suggesting that millions of individuals worldwide may have developed thyroid issues as a result of mRNA vaccinations.[53]

Neuropsychiatric Disorders

This study explored neuropsychiatric risks of mRNA COVID-19 vaccines using VAERS data (1990–2024). Compared to influenza and other vaccines, COVID-19 vaccines showed significant safety signals for cognitive impairment, psychiatric illness, and suicide/homicide, with Proportional Reporting Ratios (PRRs) far exceeding CDC/FDA thresholds, suggesting urgent need for a global vaccination moratorium.[54]

Conclusion

COVID-19 vaccines represent the most alarming scientific and regulatory failure since the earliest smallpox vaccines (which caused smallpox among other diseases). A novel technology (mRNA platform vaccines) was rushed to market to address an overhyped public health panic. There was inadequate regulatory oversight, manufacturing deficiencies, contaminated products, insufficient preclinical testing, rushed clinical trials, suppression of post-release adverse events, and continued promotion by the government of a clearly defective product. The level of regulatory malfeasance is astonishing.

Manufacturers and the CDC assert that mRNA vaccines provide protection against severe illness, hospitalization, and death, despite the failure of extensive Pfizer and Moderna trials to demonstrate such protection. Multiple studies demonstrate significant adverse events for several years following vaccination, including a rise in cancer rates.

It is worth noting that Pfizer, the leading manufacturer of COVID-19 vaccines worldwide recently acquired Seagen, a biotechnology company specializing in cancer treatments, for $43 billion.[55] What does Pfizer know about the cancer market that the public doesn't?

All COVID-19 vaccines should be immediately withdrawn from the market. At minimum, COVID-19 vaccine package inserts should contain a black box warning for risk of cardiac injury and death.

Chapter Summary

Section	Key Themes	Summary Points
Introduction	Overview of COVID-19 vaccines and regulatory issues	• Focuses on mRNA vaccines (Pfizer-BioNTech's Comirnaty, Moderna's Spikevax, mNEXSPIKE) and Novavax's protein subunit vaccine (Nuvaxovid, Covovax). • Critiques the regulatory framework for lacking placebo-controlled, randomized trials, highlighting inadequate oversight.
COVID-19	SARS-CoV-2 characteristics and vulnerable populations	• SARS-CoV-2 spreads via respiratory droplets, causing fever, cough, and shortness of breath. • Seniors (≥65 years) with comorbidities (e.g., obesity, diabetes, heart disease) face higher risks of severe illness, atypical symptoms (e.g., confusion), and long-term complications (e.g., cognitive dysfunction, organ damage).

Section	Key Themes	Summary Points
Vaccines	Vaccine types, manufacturing, and concerns	• Pfizer-BioNTech (Comirnaty): mRNA vaccine (30 mcg, ages 12+), produced using E. coli bioreactors; concerns about plasmid DNA contamination. • Moderna (Spikevax, mNEXSPIKE): mRNA vaccines (50 mcg and 10 mcg, respectively); mNEXSPIKE name raises concerns due to "Nex" (Latin for death/slaughter). • Novavax (Nuvaxovid, Covovax): Spike protein-based subunit vaccine, uses moth cells and Matrix-M adjuvant from soapbark tree extract.
New Regulatory Framework	FDA's revised vaccine approval standards	• Public vaccine uptake low: <25% of Americans got 2023–2024 boosters; <10% of children vaccinated. • FDA's new framework assumes all adults ≥65 need annual vaccination, relying on immunogenicity (antibody levels) rather than placebo-controlled trials. • For ages 6 months–64 years with risk factors, effectiveness is presumed without robust evidence. • Healthy individuals (6 months–64 years) may be subject to manufacturer-led trials, raising bias concerns.
CDC 2025 Risk Conditions	Criteria for vaccination eligibility	• Conditions include asthma, cancer, chronic kidney/lung/liver diseases, diabetes, heart conditions, HIV, mental health disorders, obesity, pregnancy, and more. • Up to 200 million Americans eligible, potentially facing pressure from healthcare providers to vaccinate.
Vaccine Schedule	2024–2025 dosing guidelines	• Ages 12–64 (at-risk): 1 dose of Spikevax, Comirnaty, or Novavax (2 doses if unvaccinated, 3–8 weeks apart). • Ages ≥65: 2 doses, 6 months apart (minimum 2 months). • mNEXSPIKE: Pending 2025 release for high-risk adults, single dose, subject to further studies.

(continued . . .)

Section	Key Themes	Summary Points
VRBPAC Approval	2025–2026 vaccine strain selection	• May 2025: VRBPAC endorsed monovalent JN.1-lineage (LP.8.1 strain) vaccine for 2025–2026. • Relies on immunogenicity data, criticized by Schaffer et al. (2025) study for undermining booster necessity.
Vaccine Effectiveness	Challenges and evidence gaps	• SARS-CoV-2's rapid mutation (e.g., Omicron subvariants NB.1.8.1, KP.3.1.1, XEC) makes vaccines outdated. • Pfizer/Moderna 2020 trials (Wuhan-Hu-1 strain) claimed 95%/94% efficacy (RRR), but ARR was 0.8% (Pfizer, NNT=125) and 1.2% (Moderna, NNT=83). • No evidence of efficacy against severe illness, hospitalization, or death. • Cleveland Clinic study showed negative efficacy (more vaccinations, higher infection risk). • 2024–2025 vaccines (targeting KP.2) rely on antibody studies, not clinical trials, with unknown efficacy against current strains.
Vaccine Safety	Adverse events and risks	• Common reactions: Fatigue (38–54%), headache (31–48%), muscle/joint pain, fever, chills, injection site pain (up to 75%). • Serious adverse events: Myocarditis, heart failure, stroke, blood clots, autoimmune diseases, neurological issues, reproductive harm, immune suppression, possible cancer promotion, out-of-hospital cardiac arrest. • mNEXSPIKE safety unverified due to lack of placebo-controlled trials. • Studies (e.g., Hulscher et al., 2024) link mRNA vaccines to increased mortality (e.g., 1,236% surge in cardiopulmonary deaths in King County, WA). • Lipid nanoparticles (LNPs) distribute systemically, crossing blood-brain barrier and placenta, causing widespread tissue damage.

Section	Key Themes	Summary Points
Specific Safety Concerns	Key studies on adverse events	• Increased mortality: Hulscher et al. (2024): 73.9% of post-vaccination deaths vaccine-related; Levi et al. (2025): Pfizer vaccine linked to 36% higher all-cause mortality. • AESIs: Myocarditis (+510%), heart attacks (+286%), strokes (+240%), Guillain-Barré syndrome (+149%). • Cancer risks: McKernan (2024): Plasmid DNA/SV40 in cancer biopsy; Alden et al. (2022): mRNA reverse-transcribed into DNA in liver cells. • Immune dysregulation: Yale study (2024): T-cell exhaustion (VAIDS), persistent spike protein (up to 709 days), EBV reactivation. • Vascular damage: Spike protein in 43.8% of mRNA-vaccinated stroke patients, persisting 17 months. • Thyroid disorders: 30% increased risk post-vaccination. • Neuropsychiatric disorders: VAERS data show elevated risks of cognitive impairment, psychiatric illness, suicide/homicide.
Conclusion	Regulatory failures and recommendations	• mRNA vaccines are criticized as a rushed, defective technology with inadequate testing and oversight. • Serious adverse events, including death, cardiac injury, and cancer risks, persist years post-vaccination. • Calls for immediate market withdrawal and black box warnings for cardiac injury risks. • Regulatory malfeasance and reliance on immunogenicity over clinical evidence undermine public trust.

CHAPTER 6

mRNA Vaccines: Warp Speed Trojan Horse

"The next step is [to halt] the mRNA platform itself . . . the manufacturer has no idea what dose they're giving, no idea where it goes in the body, and whether they are producing off-target antigens."
—NIH Director Dr. Jay Bhattacharya[1]

Found in every cell of the human body, mRNA's (messenger RNA) job is to communicate messages, or code, from DNA in a cell's nucleus to the cell's protein manufacturing system. A cell's nucleus is unimaginably complex. It hosts around twenty-five thousand segments of DNA, called genes, that are responsible for the genetic code that makes over a hundred thousand proteins essential for life.

Messenger RNA translates commands from the nucleus thousands of times a day, and after delivering its instructions, it's immediately broken down and recycled to form the next distinct mRNA genetic code, as instructed by the cell's DNA inside the nucleus.

Before 2021, few people were familiar with the concept of an mRNA vaccine. As it became better known during the COVID-19 pandemic, most thought of it as a step forward in the ongoing and inevitable march of science.

Modelled on Viruses

The idea of an mRNA vaccine comes from ancient foes: viruses like influenza, polio, and the common cold. These viruses cannot replicate on their own, so they have to find a host to supply all the ingredients they lack. Once viruses infect the body, they insidiously hijack a cell's protein-making machinery by inserting their own RNA or DNA into an unsuspecting cell, thereby creating billions of replicas of themselves.

As the newly born viruses burst forth from infected cells, the immune system attacks and destroys them—but usually not before the virus has been transmitted to other people.

The mRNA vaccines work similarly. They insert their own genetic code into a cell and force it to produce not a whole virus but a single viral protein component. The goal is for the resulting proteins to sensitize the immune system to fight future attacks of a virus containing the same protein structure.

How Are mRNA Vaccines Different from Traditional Vaccines?

Whereas mRNA vaccines take over a cell to produce a single viral protein component, most other vaccines include weakened or killed viruses or bacteria. Some use recombinant technology to produce an antigen similar to the original virus to stimulate an immune response to the target pathogen. Recombinant viral vaccines are created by inserting genes from a virus into a host species (often yeast or bacteria) to produce a component of the virus that will serve as the antigen in the vaccine. In other words, the process uses the protein-making machinery of billions of yeast or bacterial cells to make the desired antigens for vaccine production.

Prior to the mRNA vaccine, the FDA has never, in its entire history, authorized a vaccine that takes over a human cell's protein manufacturing process to produce a protein alien to the cell. This is a clearcut alteration of normal, cellular gene expression. Call it what it is: genetic manipulation or "gene therapy."

Strong objection has been made to calling mRNA vaccines gene therapy.[2] But Pfizer itself, one of two makers of mRNA COVID-19 vaccines, has said that mRNA technology is a good fit for gene editing, which means of course that the technology can be used to modify the expression of human DNA.[3]

Viruses have scores of antigens that the immune system recognizes in order to develop an effective and lasting immune response. Vaccines made up of weakened or killed viruses contain all or most of the original viral antigens. As a rule of thumb, the greater the number of antigens presented by a vaccine, the more complete and lasting the immune protection. However, current mRNA vaccines produce only a *single* protein antigen.

Why Natural Immunity Is Best

Infection produces robust and durable immunity.

Both the innate (rapid response) immune system and the adaptive (long-term memory) immune system are activated by infection, and both are essential for locking in the capacity to fight off future infections.

On the other hand, immunity trained by a vaccine with a single or limited set of antigens, like the mRNA vaccine, may be caught flat-footed when variants of the original infection are encountered. Such was the case with SARS-CoV-2 when the original vaccine based on the Wuhan strain could only mount a limited and short-lived neutralizing immune response to Omicron variants.

Viral Immune Escape

There is growing evidence that mass COVID-19 mRNA vaccination may be generating novel and potentially more virulent versions of SARS-CoV-2. In his book, *The Inescapable Immune Escape Pandemic*, Geert Vanden Bossche explains how repeated administration of mRNA COVID-19 vaccines can lead to vaccine breakthrough infections or VBTIs.[4]

VBTIs refer to cases where individuals who have been vaccinated against a disease, such as COVID-19, still become infected with the virus. Specifically, mutated regions of the SARS-CoV-2 spike (S) protein in new variants may reduce the effectiveness of antibodies generated by prior vaccination or infection, leading to breakthrough infections. This phenomenon could explain why some studies have indicated negative vaccine efficacy, where increased vaccination correlates with a higher likelihood of infection.[5]

modRNA—It Was Never mRNA

As noted, mRNA is the highly efficient messenger system used by cells to produce proteins. mRNA is a single use system; once the coded protein is made, enzymes in the cell rapidly degrade the messenger RNA into its component parts, and it is then ready to be reassembled into a new strand of mRNA as needed.

Prompt breakdown of mRNA was the basis for the often-repeated phrase that mRNA in the COVID-19 vaccine rapidly disappears after it delivers instructions for the manufacture of Spike protein.

Most people, including many health-care providers, are unaware that COVID-19 vaccines don't actually contain mRNA but a modified version known as modRNA.

modRNA Made to be Stealthy and Durable

Just four molecules called nucleotides comprise all the genetic code carried by RNA. Variations in the length and sequence of these four molecules in mRNA set the code to determine which proteins are made.

However, BioNTech/Pfizer and Moderna modified the RNA code for the Spike protein by swapping out one of the naturally occurring nucleosides (uridine) and substituting a synthetic version called pseudouridine (officially N1-methylpseudouridine). Hence, modified RNA or modRNA.

Pfizer Confirms Use of modRNA

Although it takes some digging to find amidst all the mRNA hype, the use of modRNA is confirmed by Pfizer on its website:

> [T]he Pfizer-BioNTech COVID-19 vaccine, utilizes modRNA. modRNA stands for nucleoside-modified messenger RNA and in the synthesis of the RNA used in this vaccine platform, some nucleosides, which are important biological molecules that constitute DNA and RNA, are replaced by modified nucleosides to help ***enhance immune evasion*** and protein production [emphasis ours].[6]

Does modRNA Ever Go Away?

Enhance immune evasion indeed. The effect of a substitution for one of mRNA's nucleotides is profound. Swapping pseudouridine for uridine causes modRNA to resist the expected rapid enzymatic breakdown seen with mRNA. The substitute molecule also shields modRNA from immune system attack, prolonging its life in circulation throughout the body.

This immune evasion is proving to be very successful—perhaps too successful. One study found modRNA and Spike protein hiding out in lymph nodes weeks after injection, not rapidly breaking down as promoted by the CDC and manufacturers.[7]

It is not known if modRNA ever completely clears from the body, continuing to generate toxic Spike proteins that no longer confer protection against SARS-CoV-2 variants.

An August 2023 study found Spike protein in the blood, saliva, urine, and lung fluids of people six months post–COVID-19 vaccine, suggesting mRNA may persist in some cells for extended periods of time or the body has trouble clearing excess spike proteins, or perhaps both.[8]

A report from researchers from Yale University found the presence of spike proteins and markers of altered immune function in patients with post-vaccination syndrome up to 709 days post-vaccination.[9]

As discussed in Chapter 5, spike proteins are extremely toxic to the lining of blood vessels and multiple organ systems, including the brain, heart, lungs, and blood. Their continued production due to the elusiveness of modRNA may underlie the large number of well-documented COVID-19 severe adverse events.

Spike Protein Persistence in Previously Vaccinated Patients

A 2023 paper by McCullough and colleagues suggests that SARS-CoV-2 spike proteins from infection or mRNA vaccines may remain in the body and potentially cause health issues. They propose that prolonged spike protein production, due to vaccine mRNA stabilized with pseudouridine, could explain high antibody levels months or years after vaccination.[10]

Measurement of Spike Protein Antibody Levels

There are no direct measurements of spike proteins in the body. The next best method for determining spike protein levels is to measure spike antibody levels in the blood. At least one reference laboratory, LabCorp, offers a spike antibody test patients can self-order (https://www.ondemand.labcorp.com/lab-tests/covid-19-antibody-test). The test provides a semi-quantitative measure of spike protein levels in the blood. Specifically, it detects antibodies to SARS-CoV-2 spike protein receptor binding domain, a critical component enabling viral entry into host cells.

LabCorp's test reporting range is 0.8–25,000 U/mL (units per milliliter of blood serum), with values above 25,000 U/mL reported as >25,000 U/mL. A result of ≥0.8 U/mL is considered positive, indicating detectable antibodies to the SARS-CoV-2 spike protein, suggestive of prior infection or vaccination.

Spike Antibody Results in Clinical Practice

Mary Talley Bowden, MD, a physician practicing in Texas who has cared for hundreds of COVID-19 vaccine-injured patients, has made numerous posts on X.com (@MDBreathe) about her patients' spike antibody test results.

For example, in a post in May 2025, she reported elevated spike protein antibody levels in vaccinated patients (mean: 13,183–13,427, range: 335–>25,000) compared to unvaccinated patients (mean: 865–1,323, range: 3.2–9,438).[11]

These results are consistent with findings by other physician colleagues. The question remains—can anything be done to reduce the amount of residual spike protein?

Spike Detoxification Protocols

It is unclear whether spike proteins can be degraded in the body and whether doing so will result in mitigation of post-vaccine injuries or prevent future injury. If persistent spike protein elevation is due to continued production by residual modRNA, then clearance of spike protein may only lead to more spike production.

One approach to spike detoxification was reported by McCullough and colleagues in the paper cited above.[12] Their Base Spike Detoxification protocol, published in the *Journal of American Physicians and Surgeons,* recommends several supplements to degrade spike protein and reduce inflammation.

Other detoxification protocols have been published by the Independent Medical Alliance.[13] These include a variety of modalities and include use of off label prescription medications, medical supplements, photo biomodulation, intermittent fasting, and hyperbaric oxygen, among others.

Research into the implications of persistent elevation of spike protein antibodies and the effectiveness of detoxification measures is urgently needed.

Does mRNA Integrate into the Human Genome?

One of the many assurances offered the public about the safety of COVID-19 mRNA vaccines is that they would not integrate into and potentially alter the human genome. Pfizer has made considerable effort to paint any information to the contrary as "misinformation and disinformation."

Pfizer's website "The Facts" under the section "Does an mRNA vaccine change your DNA?" states unequivocally:

> No, mRNA vaccines do not alter your DNA. In fact, they don't interact directly with your DNA at all.[14]

Pfizer's assertion references an article from 2023 titled, "The evolution of SARS-CoV-2" as evidence for the lack of genetic alteration.[15]

A review of that paper reveals it has no relevance whatsoever to whether mRNA injections alter DNA or interact with the genome. Rather, the article examines the factors that may explain how the virus has evolved into new variants and the selective forces that likely drove the evolution of higher transmissibility.

In contrast, as of publication four independent sources have demonstrated a COVID-19 vaccine mRNA-host DNA interaction.[16]

Study	Key Findings	Source
InModia Lab[17] (Germany)	Detected vaccine-derived spike protein, mRNA, and SV40 promoter/enhancer sequences in human tissue samples years after the final injection, suggesting long-term persistence and possible genomic integration.	https://inmodia.de/en /services/detection-of -spike-protein/

(continued . . .)

Study	Key Findings	Source
Neo7Bioscience + University of North Texas[18]	Using the REViSS platform, found evidence of reverse transcription, synthetic mRNA persistence, and gene dysregulation in vaccinated individuals, with downregulated tumor suppressor genes (e.g., TP53, BRCA1/2), upregulated oncogenic signaling, and elevated molecular instability scores compared to controls.	Hulscher, N. BREAKING—Reverse Transcription, Abnormal Gene Expression Detected in Patients After mRNA Vaccination.
Kyriakopoulos et al.[19]	Demonstrated mRNA integration into the human genome via LINE-1 retrotransposition, Polymerase theta (Polθ), and defective DNA repair mechanisms, potentially leading to cancer, autoimmunity, or inheritable genetic damage.	Kyriakopoulos, A. M. (2022). Potential mechanisms for human genome integration of genetic code from SARS-CoV-2 mRNA vaccination: Implications for disease. *Journal of Clinical Immunology and Immunotherapy*
Aldén, et al.[20]	Demonstrated that Pfizer's BNT162b2 mRNA is reverse-transcribed into DNA in human liver cells within six hours.	Intracellular Reverse Transcription of Pfizer BioNTech COVID-19 mRNA Vaccine BNT162b2 In Vitro in Human Liver Cell Line. *Current Issues in Molecular Biology.* 2022

modRNA Causes Junk Protein Production

The substitution of pseudouridine for natural uridine in modRNA has another potentially dangerous consequence. As modRNA translates its genetic code to the protein manufacturing systems inside a cell, the presence of pseudouridine occasionally triggers a glitch in reading the code, referred to as "frameshifting."[21]

A 2023 study published in *Nature* found that modRNA vaccines containing pseudouridine can cause ribosomal frameshifting. This occurs when ribosomes misread the mRNA sequence, shifting the reading frame and producing aberrant or "junk" proteins.[22]

Junk protein is just that, a protein that has no function yet may be viewed by the immune system as a foreign invader that needs to be destroyed. The subsequent immune reaction may be inflammatory and potentially exacerbates the known toxicity of modRNA in the vaccinated.

Researchers at Cambridge University recently confirmed that 25 to 30 percent of patients who received the Pfizer mRNA vaccine experienced an unintended immune response in the form of antibody production against frameshifted spike proteins. This means that vaccinated persons are forming antibodies against random proteins caused by frameshifting, which can lead to an unwanted inflammatory response including an autoimmune reaction.[23]

NIH Director Bhattacharya criticizes mRNA vaccines for their unpredictability. He states, "The dose of the antigen . . . could be one or two, three, five. There's no control over it," noting variable antigen production and biodistribution throughout the body.[24]

Director Bhattacharya adds, "mRNA technology is not perfect . . . you often get antigens . . . not in the code itself" due to frameshifting, raising regulatory concerns about dosing, distribution, and protein fidelity, as these factors remain uncontrollable.[25]

A Contaminated Vaccine

Drug manufacturers and regulatory agencies have insisted for the past five years that the COVID-19 vaccines were safe. Independent scientists, including Health Canada, however, have reported Pfizer's mRNA vaccine to be contaminated.[26, 27, 28]

Contaminants consist of DNA plasmids, which are circular strands of DNA left over from the production process (described below in Process 1 and Process 2). In a published scientific paper, DNA contamination was reported to be well above allowable limits in vials tested.[29]

Unexpected DNA contamination averaged over 100 percent, resulting in more DNA than mRNA in Pfizer's shot. Moderna's vaccine ran about 50 percent contamination.[30] In addition, the researchers found up to 186 billion copies of the SV40 cancer promoter gene sequences and virus spike protein in the DNA contaminant.[31] SV40 poses a risk of permanently altering human DNA.

Perhaps most alarming is that contaminated vaccine batches correlated with VAERS serious adverse event reports, suggesting the potential harm of mRNA vaccine contamination is more than theoretical.

The scientists concluded that "these data demonstrate the presence of billions to hundreds of billions of DNA molecules per dose in these vaccines" and that "all products tested exceeded the guidelines for residual DNA set by the FDA and WHO by 188 to 509-fold. Our findings extend existing concerns about vaccine safety.[32]

Process 1 and Process 2

The reason for the contamination appears to be that a different manufacturing process was used for vaccine mass production (Process 2) than was used to make vaccines for the clinical trials (Process 1). As will be discussed, Process 2 more readily lends itself to contamination.

The existence of two separate processes was not known until the summer of 2022 when two Israeli researchers noticed that Pfizer amended its clinical trial protocol, referring to Process 1 and Process 2.[33]

Subsequently, in 2023 a pharmacist was tasked by the court system to review documents a judge forced Pfizer to disclose (documents the company intended to shield from public view for seventy-five years). The pharmacist found that Pfizer had conducted a smaller trial within their major study. The majority of patients received a vaccine made with Process 1. However, some patients were given vaccines from a different manufacturing process, Process 2, without being informed. The processes turned out to be quite different, with Process 2 showing evidence of considerable contamination.[34]

Manufacturing Process 1, deployed by Pfizer to make the COVID vaccine for the clinical trial, used a process akin to a photocopier (polymerase chain reaction, or PCR), making multiple clones of the original mRNA. The PCR process is very precise, but it is expensive and difficult to commercially scale up to produce billions of doses.

Significantly, Pfizer's entire pivotal clinical trial, except for about 250 participants, received Process 1-derived mRNA vaccine.[35] Subsequent to the clinical trial, all vaccines were produced by a different process referred to as Process 2, which has been claimed to result in substantial contamination of vaccine batches.

Process 2 employs a completely different manufacturing process, one that uses *E. coli* bacteria to produce mRNA in large batches capable of making millions of doses at a time. Unfortunately, during Process 2, DNA left over from the genetically manipulated E. coli can contaminate the final product, which is what happened in this case, hence the DNA plasmid fragments found by the independent researchers noted above, which also happened to contain SV40 genetic material.

A 2023 Ontario study found billions of DNA molecules per dose in Pfizer-BioNTech and Moderna vaccines, exceeding FDA/WHO guidelines by 188–509-fold. Process 2's plasmid amplification introduced complex DNA fragments, raising purity and long-term safety concerns as vaccination campaigns continue.[36]

The bait and switch from Process 1 to Process 2 should have been disclosed to the public. Moreover, since the FDA knew of the two separate manufacturing processes, they should have required a separate, randomized, controlled clinical trial using vaccine from Process 2 before authorizing its release. Instead, the FDA accepted a secret, limited clinical trial of just 250 patients, insufficient to detect safety signals or to establish effectiveness.

Key Differences Between Process 1 and Process 2

Aspect	Process 1 (Clinical Trials)	Process 2 (Mass Production)
Scale	Small-scale, limited batches for trials	Large-scale, millions of doses (~3.6M doses/batch)
mRNA Integrity	Higher (~90–100%) due to rigorous purification	Lower (~70–90%) due to scaled-up, less stringent methods
Purification	Extensive, manual, high-purity methods	Streamlined, automated for higher throughput
LNP Encapsulation	Small-scale, controlled mixing systems	Multiple parallel microfluidic jet mixers for rapid scaling
Production Speed	Slower, quality-focused	Faster, volume-focused
Testing in Trials	Used for nearly all trial participants (~43,000)	Tested on ~250 participants before public rollout
Facilities	Primarily Andover, Mainz, Kalamazoo, Puurs	Expanded global network (20+ sites, 300+ suppliers)
Adverse Events	Lower reported rates in trials	Higher rates (1.5–3x) in some analyses post-crossover

sa-mRNA

Researchers have developed another version of modified RNA, something called self-amplifying or sa-mRNA that replicates its own modRNA once inside the cell (also referred to as replicon mRNA). The first such self-copying RNA vaccine for COVID-19 won full approval in late 2023 in Japan.[37]

Using a person's own cells as a factory, sa-mRNA continues production of antigens on its own. In theory, a smaller dose of sa-mRNA would be needed to produce the equivalent amount of protein as higher doses of modRNA. However, even sa-mRNA is limited to a single antigen per vaccine, regardless of the amount.

However, sa-mRNA raises alarming questions. How does sa-mRNA know when to shut itself off? Does potential overproduction of a single antigen excessively focus the immune response (i.e., immune imprinting, as discussed below), thereby compromising immune response to future variants? sa-mRNA's replication can strain cellular resources, as it generates many RNA copies and proteins, potentially disrupting normal cell functions, especially in sensitive cells. Another concern is the potential for autoimmune disorders as a result of immune hyperstimulation.

Risks Related to Self-Amplification May Far Outweigh Any Possible Benefits

In a Phase 1 trial in Uganda, a COVID-19 replicon or sa-mRNA injection was given to forty-two healthy adults.[38] The results were alarming: thirty-nine Grade

3 or higher hematological adverse events occurred after the second dose, affecting 93 percent of participants. Grade 3 events are severe, often requiring clinical intervention. Common abnormalities included:

- **Thrombocytopenia** (low platelet count, internal bleeding risk)
- **Lymphopenia** (suppressed adaptive immune response)
- **Neutropenia** (lowered neutrophils, increasing infection risk)

Additionally, 85.4 percent experienced systemic adverse events such as muscle pain, joint pain, vomiting, and fever. Laboratory abnormalities worsened after the second dose, suggesting cumulative toxicity or immune priming. These events affected healthy adults.

Although the data showed otherwise, the authors called the vaccine "well tolerated."[39]

FDA Fast-Tracks Replicon mRNA for Bird Flu

The same sa-mRNA platform used in the Uganda study is now being deployed for H5N1 bird flu vaccines. FDA authorized a Phase 1 trial in 2024 by Arcturus Therapeutics that is backed by the Gates Foundation ($1 million) and the Biomedical Advanced Research and Development Authority or BARDA[40] ($63 million). Arcturus developed the first approved sa-mRNA COVID-19 vaccine in Japan in 2023.

The trial compares two different doses of the Arcturus vaccine (ARCT-2304) with a first-generation mRNA vaccine. Absence of a true placebo immediately raises questions about trial safety controls. Two features about the vaccine used in the trial are novel.

The first is the sa-mRNA encodes for two separate proteins. To date, sa-mRNA vaccines have only encoded for a single protein, the S or spike protein. The Arcturus vaccine encodes for two different proteins, the S or spike protein and the N or nucleocapsid protein. This has a theoretical benefit of better training the immune system to identify the virus but also raises concerns about systemic side effects and immune disorders as a result of dispersion of these foreign proteins throughout the body (recall, they don't just stick around at the injection site).

Second, a novel lipid nanoparticle encapsulates the sa-mRNA. The LUNAR® lipid nanoparticle (LNP) used in Arcturus Therapeutics' ARCT-2304 H5N1 self-amplifying mRNA (sa-mRNA) vaccine differs from the LNPs used in Pfizer-BioNTech's Comirnaty and Moderna's Spikevax mRNA vaccines in composition, manufacturing, stability, and functional properties. These differences stem from the unique requirements of saRNA (which amplifies RNA in cells) versus conventional mRNA.

The absence of a true placebo in the clinical trial, encoding two separate proteins, and a completely novel LNP make it essential to carefully measure safety endpoints, reactogenicity (adverse physical reactions), and immune response as measured by antibody levels. Failure to measure actual disease endpoints (infection, hospitalization, severe disease, etc.) further undermines confidence in the clinical trial.

modRNA Vaccines in the Pipeline

The FDA remains enamored with mRNA vaccines. The technology enables rapid prototyping of custom-tailored antigens using recombinant DNA technology that inserts a cloned (copied) gene into a bacterial cell to produce a desired gene product such as modRNA. The process is also used to make therapies such as insulin and growth hormone.

FDA shares manufacturers' enthusiasm for the rapidity of development and cost-effectiveness of the large-batch, plasmid-based, manufacturing process.

Consequently, FDA has recently (as of publication) granted fast-track designation to three vaccines. Fast-track designation expedites development and review for vaccines, addressing what FDA considers to be serious conditions or unmet medical needs. These designations should raise alarm with the public as there is no evidence that current public health measures are insufficient to control and treat these conditions.

Vaccines Granted Fast-Track Designation

Date of Designation	Company	Vaccine Candidate	FDA Fast Track Designation Details
Dec 11, 2024	Sanofi	Influenza + COVID-19 Combination Vaccines (with Novavax)	Two candidates combining Sanofi's Fluzone High-Dose or Flublok with Novavax's adjuvanted COVID-19 vaccine for adults ≥50 years.
Mar 26, 2025	Sanofi	Chlamydia mRNA Vaccine	mRNA-based vaccine targeting chlamydia, aimed at addressing unmet medical needs for this infection.
Apr 10, 2025	Arcturus	ARCT-2304 (sa-mRNA Influenza H5N1)	Self-amplifying mRNA vaccine for H5N1 influenza, designed for lower doses and enhanced immune response.

At least four mRNA flu vaccines have begun clinical trials, including those from Pfizer, Moderna, Sanofi, and the National Institute for Allergies and Infectious Diseases (NIAID).

For example, Moderna is developing modRNA vaccines for respiratory syncytial virus (RSV), Zika virus, HIV, Cytomegalovirus (CMV), COVID-19, influenza, and a combination COVID-19/Influenza vaccine.

In addition to influenza mRNA vaccines, Pfizer is working on a shingles vaccine and combination COVID-19/RSV and COVID-19/Influenza vaccines.

mRNA Vaccines in Late Stages of Development

As of the latest available data, several mRNA vaccines for infectious diseases are in Phase 2 or greater clinical trials. This means they could become commercialized in the next year or so.

The table below includes both non-replicating mRNA and self-amplifying RNA (saRNA) vaccines.

mRNA Vaccines for Infectious Diseases in Phase 2 or Greater Clinical Trials

Vaccine Candidate	Developer	Target Disease	Clinical Trial Phase	ClinicalTrials. gov ID	Notes
mRNA-1647	Moderna	Cytomegalovirus (CMV)	Phase 2/3	NCT05683457, NCT05085366	Encodes CMV pentamer complex and glycoprotein B antigens
mRNA-1010	Moderna	Seasonal Influenza	Phase 3	NCT04956575, NCT05415462	Quadrivalent vaccine targeting WHO-proposed strains
mRNA-1083	Moderna	Influenza/ COVID-19 Combination	Phase 3	Not specified	Combines flu and COVID-19 protection
mRNA-1403	Moderna	Norovirus	Phase 3	Not specified	Targets multiple norovirus strains
Quadrivalent modRNA	Pfizer	Seasonal Influenza	Phase 3	NCT05540522	Targets four influenza strains

Vaccine Candidate	Developer	Target Disease	Clinical Trial Phase	ClinicalTrials.gov ID	Notes
ARCoV	Abogen (China)	COVID-19	Phase 3	Not specified	Safe, induces high neutralizing antibody titers
mRNA-1975/ mRNA-1982	Moderna	Lyme Disease	Phase 2	NCT05975099	Encodes outer surface protein A (OspA)
mRNA-1345	Moderna	Respiratory Syncytial Virus (RSV)	Phase 2/3	NCT05127434	Targets older adults (60+)
mRNA-1893	Moderna	Zika Virus	Phase 2	NCT04917861	Encodes Zika virus antigens
mRNA-1073	Moderna	Influenza/ COVID-19 Combination	Phase 2	Not specified	Combined protection for flu and COVID-19
BNT163	BioNTech	Herpes Simplex Virus 2 (HSV-2)	Phase 2	NCT05432583	Targets genital herpes lesions

It's for Your "Convenience"

Combination vaccines are promoted for their convenience by minimizing the number of injections. However, they restrict choice when offered in combination and make full disclosure of benefits and risks of each separate vaccine more difficult. They are also a mechanism by which pharmaceutical companies can boost sales.

The industry is concerned about the steep drop-off in sales following record profits from COVID-19 vaccines.[41] It seems public appetite for the relatively ineffective and potentially quite harmful vaccines has waned.

Vaccine manufacturers hope that by combining an established and generally accepted yearly shot like influenza vaccine with a vaccine whose sales are lagging, overall sales will pick back up.

As the president of Pfizer remarked recently during an investors call, he believes the convenience of offering combination vaccines will "unlock a significant potential by improving vaccination rates."[42]

Significant potential for whom?

Look for many new combination vaccines in the years to come to boost corporate bottom lines. Most of these products will use modRNA or sa-mRNA technologies and will be pitched to consumers as a convenience that unlocks "significant potential," but perhaps not human potential.

Lipid Nanoparticles (LNPs)

LNPs are essential to deliver modRNA and sa-mRNA to the cells, but are they safe?

On its own, modRNA containing the genetic code for a particular protein has difficulty passing through cell walls. For modRNA to produce the desired protein, it must enter the cell and take control of its protein manufacturing apparatus. A delivery system is essential to carry modRNA to the cell surface and facilitate uptake and release of modRNA inside the cell.

LNPs were selected by researchers to encapsulate modRNA because of their ability to evade immune system attack and efficiency at passing through cell membranes. They are, for all intents and purposes, a molecular Trojan horse. LNPs can even penetrate blood vessel–organ interfaces usually resistant to vaccines or even viruses, such as the blood-brain barrier and the placenta.

Unfortunately, LNPs are toxic and can trigger inflammatory-related adverse events and anaphylaxis.

Back in the 1990s when mRNA platform technology was being developed, one of the inventors, Robert Malone, MD, abandoned LNPs due to their toxicity.[43] This lesson appears lost on Malone's successors, who continued the development of mRNA applications using LNPs.

One such successor was Stéphane Bancel, CEO of Moderna, who stated in 2016:

> "Delivery—actually getting RNA into cells—has long bedeviled the whole field. On their own, RNA molecules have a hard time reaching their targets. They work better if they're wrapped up in a delivery mechanism, such as nanoparticles made of lipids. But those nanoparticles can lead to dangerous side effects, especially if a patient has to take repeated doses over months or years."[44]

Despite these concerns, Moderna joined Pfizer as one of the first two manufacturers of COVID-19 mRNA vaccines that used lipid nanoparticle carriers.

Vaccine manufacturers have now conceded that the carrier technology used by their vaccines can be toxic. A paper published in 2024 by Moderna scientists found that the lipid nanoparticles used in its COVID-19 mRNA vaccine can be toxic and might be the root cause of many of the side effects experienced by people post vaccination.[45] These include, according to the authors, "heart inflammation and severe allergic shock, . . . most likely triggered by PEGylated lipid nanoparticles."

As noted below, PEG is polyethylene glycol which can be highly reactogenic (can cause adverse immune reactions).

LNP Toxicity

LNPs are known to be toxic to DNA through the release of reactive oxygen molecules that penetrate the cell nucleus.[46] The particles are coated with polyethylene glycol (PEG), which helps to stabilize the LNPs and keeps them from clumping. However, PEG can trigger anaphylactic allergic reaction, GI distress, electrolyte imbalances, and can be neurotoxic.[47]

LNPs are also known to activate the complement (inflammatory) system and stimulate the secretion of pro-inflammatory cytokines.[48] Complement and cytokines are part of the innate or immediate response component of the immune system. Overstimulation from LNPs can precipitate an overly aggressive immune response that can result in life-threatening side effects.

Several studies describe inflammatory-related adverse events following modRNA injections, including stroke, pericarditis, and myocarditis.[49, 50, 51]

LNPs are widely distributed

Despite what the public was told about the COVID-19 vaccination staying in the arm and rapidly breaking down, LNPs disperse throughout the body within hours of injection.

Pfizer knew this in advance of FDA's Emergency Use Authorization. "In summary," Pfizer wrote about their own vaccine uptake and distribution study, "over 48 hours, the LNP distributed mainly to liver, adrenal glands, spleen and ovaries, with maximum concentrations observed at 8–48 hours post-dose."[52]

So much for modRNA vaccine injection localizing to the arm and posing no risk to other organ systems. The observation of LNPs in the reproductive system was a harbinger of the disastrous effects later observed on fertility and pregnancy (see Chapter 11: Vaccines During Pregnancy: Caveat Emptor).

The safety of LNPs as a delivery vehicle remains unproven. Clearly, more research is needed on the safety and toxicity of these compounds before their further use as a vaccine transport vehicle.

Innate (Rapid Response) & Adaptive (Memory) Immune Systems

The *innate system* identifies a foreign invader, mounts an initial defense, and calls for backup from the adaptive immune system through chemical signals. In turn, antibodies are produced specific to the antigens found on the foreign invaders, allowing for their destruction.

The *adaptive system* serves as a library of potential threats, storing the memory of previous invaders in specialized immune cells that can rapidly respond to future infections. The adaptive system is also highly flexible with built-in redundancy, responding to countless variations of previous threats.

The adaptive system can effectively respond to thousands of variants of a particular pathogen by identifying viral components that are less likely to mutate over time.

While antibody measurements are often employed as an indicator of vaccine effectiveness, evidence indicates that antibody responses do not reliably correlate with actual vaccine efficacy.

modRNA vaccine-induced immunity is directed at a single antigen. In the case of COVID-19 vaccine, this was the Spike or S protein region of the SARS-CoV-2 virus. Mutations to this region in circulating viruses help evade a sterilizing immune response to new variants from the vaccine, making reinfection more likely. This phenomenon is known as immune imprinting.

Immune Imprinting

As discussed, the adaptive immune system is a critical component of protective immunity. Exposure to a single viral antigen such as the modRNA-generated Spike protein might limit the generation of new immune responses. Essentially, new variants may be capable of evading a neutralizing immune response if protective immunity was trained on a single protein.[53]

The resulting narrowly focused immunity is referred to as immune imprinting (sometimes called original antigenic sin or OAS). OAS may result in several immune system impairments.

Immune imprinting and lack of development of neutralizing antibodies increases the infectiousness of the virus to vaccinated and boosted adults. Immune imprinting may explain why the greater the number of COVID-19 vaccinations previously received, the higher the risk of contracting COVID-19, according to a study from the Cleveland Clinic.[54]

Conclusion

modRNA vaccines are a failed technology that have not been proven safe or effective. modRNA resists natural breakdown by the immune system and can persist in the body for weeks to months or longer, generating dangerous Spike proteins. sa-mRNA vaccines pose the added risk of unlimited foreign protein production with resulting immune dysregulation and autoimmune disorders.

Quantitative spike antibody tests are now available as indirect measures of the burden of hazardous spike proteins. Various detoxification regimens have been proposed.

LNP carriers are known to be toxic and do not remain at the injection site. They disperse modRNA throughout the body, including to the reproductive organs and brain. Evidence is emerging about the long-term harms of modRNA and persistent spike protein production.

Until definitive, multi-year clinical trials demonstrate both the safety and effectiveness of modRNA and sa-mRNA vaccines compared with a true placebo, these vaccines should be withdrawn until their risk and benefits are more clearly understood.

Chapter Summary

Section	Key Points
Introduction to mRNA Basics	• mRNA, found in all human cells, translates DNA instructions into ~100,000 proteins from 25,000 genes. • mRNA delivers codes 1,000s of times daily, then breaks down and recycles; unfamiliar to public pre-2021. • Seen as a scientific advancement during COVID-19.
Modelled on Viruses	• mRNA vaccines mimic viruses (e.g., influenza, polio) that hijack cells to replicate. • Vaccines insert genetic code to produce a single viral protein, aiming to train immunity against future infections.
How Are mRNA Vaccines Different From Traditional Vaccines?	• mRNA vaccines produce a single antigen, unlike traditional vaccines (weakened/killed viruses or recombinant antigens) that expose the immune system to multiple antigens. • First FDA-authorized cell-hijacking vaccine; considered genetic manipulation, though Pfizer denies "gene therapy" label.
Why Natural Immunity Is Best	• Infection activates innate (rapid) and adaptive (long-term) immunity, offering robust, durable protection. • mRNA vaccines' single-antigen focus may fail against variants (e.g., Omicron vs. Wuhan strain).
Viral Immune Escape	• Mass mRNA vaccination may drive novel, virulent SARS-CoV-2 variants (Vanden Bossche's theory). • Vaccine breakthrough infections (VBTIs) occur due to mutated spike proteins evading antibodies, linked to negative efficacy.
modRNA - It Was Never mRNA	• COVID-19 vaccines use modRNA (modified RNA with pseudouridine replacing uridine), not natural mRNA, enhancing immune evasion and protein production. • Pfizer confirms modRNA use for immune evasion.

(continued . . .)

Section	Key Points
modRNA Made to be Stealthy and Durable	• Pseudouridine resists breakdown, prolonging modRNA/spike protein presence (weeks to months, e.g., lymph nodes, blood). • Studies (2023) show spike protein persistence (up to 709 days), linked to adverse events.
modRNA Causes Junk Protein Production	• Pseudouridine causes frameshifting, producing junk proteins; 25–30% of Pfizer recipients show unintended immune responses. • NIH's Bhattacharya highlights uncontrolled antigen production and regulatory concerns.
A Contaminated Vaccine	• Independent studies (e.g., Health Canada) found DNA contamination (100%+ in Pfizer, 50% in Moderna) exceeding FDA/WHO limits by 188–509-fold. • Contaminants include SV40, linked to higher VAERS adverse events.
Process 1 and Process 2	• Process 1 (clinical trials): Precise PCR, high purity, used for ~43,000 participants. • Process 2 (mass production): E. coli-based, contaminated with DNA plasmids, used for ~250 trial participants and public rollout. • Switch undisclosed; FDA accepted limited Process 2 trial.
Unveiling Residual DNA Concerns	• 2023 Ontario study confirms billions of DNA molecules per dose, raising purity/safety issues. • Process 2's contamination linked to adverse events; public disclosure and further trials needed.
sa-mRNA	• Self-amplifying mRNA (sa-mRNA) replicates in cells, approved in Japan (2023); risks include overproduction and immune dysregulation. • Uganda trial (2023) showed 93% severe adverse events (e.g., thrombocytopenia) post-second dose.
FDA Fast-Tracks Replicon mRNA for Bird Flu	• Arcturus' ARCT-2304 (sa-mRNA H5N1) in 2024 Phase 1 trial uses dual proteins and novel LUNAR® LNP. • No placebo, untested safety endpoints; backed by Gates/BARDA ($64M).
modRNA Vaccines in the Pipeline	• FDA's Fast Track for Sanofi (influenza/COVID, chlamydia), Arcturus (H5N1) vaccines reflects enthusiasm for rapid development. • Multiple mRNA vaccines (e.g., Moderna for RSV, HIV) in Phase 2/3 trials.
mRNA Vaccines in Late Stages of Development	• Includes Moderna (CMV, influenza, RSV), Pfizer (influenza, shingles), and others in Phase 2/3 trials. • Targets diverse diseases; commercialization possible within a year.

Section	Key Points
It's for Your 'Convenience'	• Combination vaccines (e.g., flu/COVID) boost sales but limit choice and disclosure. • Industry aims to recover from COVID-19 vaccine sales drop using convenience marketing.
Lipid Nanoparticles (LNPs)	• LNPs deliver modRNA, penetrating barriers (e.g., blood-brain, placenta); toxic, linked to inflammation (e.g., myocarditis). • Malone abandoned LNPs in 1990s; 2024 Moderna study confirms LNP toxicity (e.g., PEG reactions).
LNP Toxicity	• LNPs release reactive oxygen, damaging DNA; PEG causes anaphylaxis, neurotoxicity. • Widely distributed (liver, ovaries) within 48 hours, contradicting localized claims.
Innate & Adaptive Immune System	• Innate responds rapidly, adaptive builds memory; modRNA's limited antigens hinder variant response. • Natural immunity offers broader, cross-reactive protection.
Response to Other Viruses Affected	• Narrow immunity from modRNA reduces cross-reactivity, raising chronic infection risk. • Natural immunity builds broader defenses.
Immune Imprinting	• Single-antigen focus (e.g., Spike) causes imprinting, reducing variant response (OAS). • Cleveland Clinic study links higher vaccination to increased COVID-19 risk.
Conclusion	• modRNA/sa-mRNA unproven, persistent, and toxic; LNPs disperse widely with unknown long-term effects. • Withdraw until multi-year placebo trials confirm safety/efficacy; prioritize natural immunity.

CHAPTER 7

Shingles Vaccine:
The Emperor Still Has No Clothes

The shingles vaccine, Shingrix, is widely recommended for adults aged fifty and older to prevent herpes zoster and its complications. This chapter critically assesses its efficacy and safety, questioning whether the benefits justify the risks for healthy older adults.

Shingles

Shingles, also known as herpes zoster, is a viral infection caused by the varicella-zoster virus (VZV), the same virus that causes chickenpox. After a person recovers from chickenpox, VZV remains dormant in the body's nerve tissues. Years later, the virus can reactivate as shingles, often triggered by factors like stress, aging, a weakened immune system, or certain medications.[1]

Key Characteristics:
- Symptoms: Shingles typically presents as a painful, blistering rash on one side of the body or face, often in a band or strip along a nerve path. Other symptoms may include:
  - Burning, tingling, or itching before the rash appears
  - Fever, headache, or fatigue
  - Sensitivity to touch or severe nerve pain (postherpetic neuralgia, a potential complication)
- Duration: The rash usually lasts two to four weeks, but nerve pain can persist longer in some cases.
- Contagion: Shingles itself is not contagious, but a person with active shingles can spread VZV to someone who hasn't had chickenpox or no longer has immunity from the chickenpox vaccine (estimated ten years

or less), potentially causing chickenpox in that individual. Transmission occurs through direct contact with the rash's blisters.

- Risk Factors:
  - Age (most common in adults over 50).
  - Weakened immune system (e.g., due to HIV, cancer, or immunosuppressive drugs).
  - Previous chickenpox infection.
- Complications:
  - Postherpetic neuralgia (PHN): Persistent nerve pain after the rash heals, more common in older adults.
  - Vision loss: If shingles affect the eye (ophthalmic zoster).
  - Skin infections or, rarely, neurological issues.
- Treatment:
  - Antiviral medications (e.g., acyclovir, valacyclovir) can reduce symptom severity and duration if they start early.
  - Pain management may include over-the-counter pain relievers, topical treatments, or prescription medications for severe cases.

Approved Shingles Vaccine

The CDC recommends Shingrix® (recombinant zoster vaccine or RZV) for the prevention of herpes zoster (shingles) and related complications, including postherpetic neuralgia (PHN- persistent pain after an episode of shingles). A recombinant vaccine is a type of vaccine created using recombinant DNA technology, where inserting specific genes from a pathogen (e.g., a virus or bacterium) into a host organism (like yeast, bacteria, or mammalian cells) produces a protein or antigen. The antigen, a harmless component of the pathogen, is isolated and utilized in the vaccine to elicit an immune response without inducing the disease.

Shingrix® (GSK) Dosage

CDC recommends two doses for adults aged fifty years and older, or for adults nineteen years and older who are or will be immunodeficient or immunosuppressed (e.g., diabetic, cancer patient, steroid dependent, etc.).

Vaccine Effectiveness: Shingrix®[2]

Shingles

- CLAIM—prevention of shingles
  - 91 percent vaccine effectiveness for prevention of shingles
  - Based on Relative Risk Reduction or RRR calculation

- Actual Effectiveness
  - Absolute Risk Reduction or ARR = 0.38 percent
  - Number Needed to Treat (NNT) or number needed to be vaccinated for one person to avoid an infection = 263 (one vaccinated person out of 263 will benefit)

Post-herpetic Neuralgia (PHN)

- CLAIM—prevention of post-herpetic neuralgia
  - 85 percent vaccine effectiveness for prevention of PHN
- Actual Effectiveness
  - ARR = 0.36 percent
  - NNT = 277 (one vaccinated person out of 277 will benefit)

Vaccine Effectiveness Based on Shingrix® Package Insert

Category	Details
Shingrix®—Prevention of Shingles	**Claim:** 91% Vaccine Effectiveness for prevention of shingles based on Relative Risk Reduction (RRR) calculation
	Actual Effectiveness per patient: ARR = 0.38% **NNT** = 2625 (1 vaccinated person out of 2625 will benefit)
Shingrix®—Prevention of Post-Herpetic Neuralgia (PHN)	**Claim:** 85% Vaccine Effectiveness for prevention of PHN based on RRR
	Actual Effectiveness per patient: ARR = 0.36% **NNT** = 277 (1 vaccinated person out of 277 will benefit)
Notes: The claimed effectiveness (91% for shingles, 85% for PHN) is based on clinical trial data and reflects Relative Risk Reduction (RRR). ARR and NNT reflect real-world estimates from a patient perspective. ARR (Absolute Risk Reduction): The actual reduction in risk of shingles or PHN per patient due to the vaccine. NNT (Number Needed to Treat): The number of individuals requiring vaccination in order to prevent a single case of shingles or postherpetic neuralgia (PHN).	

Shingrix® Effectiveness Data Update

Zerbo and colleagues published an updated analysis in June 2025 of Shingrix® efficacy against Post-Herpetic Neuralgia (PHN) and Herpes Zoster Ophthalmicus (HZO–eye involvement).[3] They accumulated data from four health plans from January 1, 2018, to December 31, 2022, including adults aged fifty years or older. The overall rate was low at a cumulative 2.3% for both conditions for the nearly two million cases examined over five years.

As with many vaccine studies, reported Vaccine Effectiveness (VE) based on Relative Risk Reduction always presents a more favorable benefit profile for vaccines than is the case in practice. As found in this study, a low risk of occurrence for PHN and HZO should immediately trigger a recalculation of VE based on Absolute Risk Reduction (ARR) and Number Needed to Treat (NNT). The NNT represents the number of people who need to be vaccinated to prevent one additional case of PHN or HZO over the given time period (in this case, from thirty days post-vaccination up to one year, and from three to four years post-vaccination).

The study also found significant deterioration in vaccine effectiveness over time and if steroids had been given prior to the shots.[4]

Post-herpetic Neuralgia (PHN)
- CLAIM—Prevention of PHN
  - RRR (30 days up to 1 year)
    - 88.2% vaccine effectiveness for prevention of PHN
  - RRR (3 to 4 years)
    - 85.6% vaccine effectiveness for prevention of PHN
- Actual Effectiveness
  - 30 days post vaccination up to 1 year
    - ARR = 0.0381%
    - NNT = 2625 (1 case of PHN prevented for every 2625 vaccinations)
  - 3 to 4 years post vaccination
    - ARR = 0.037%
    - NNT = 2703 (1 case of PHN prevented for every 2703 vaccinations)

Herpes Zoster Ophthalmicus (HZO)
- CLAIM—Prevention of HZO
  - RRR (30 days up to 1 year)
    - 75.5% vaccine effectiveness for prevention of HZO

- RRR (3 to 4 years)
  - 71.2% vaccine effectiveness for prevention of HZO
- Actual Effectiveness
  - 30 days post vaccination up to 1 year
    - ARR = 0.0349%
    - NNT = 2865 (1 case of HZO prevented for every 2865 vaccinations)
  - 3 to 4 years post vaccination
    - ARR = 0.0329%
    - NNT = 3038 (1 case of HZO prevented for every 3038 vaccinations)

Vaccine Effectiveness Based on 2025 Study by Zerbo, et al.

Condition	Claim	RRR (30 days up to 1 year)	RRR (3 to 4 years)	Actual Effectiveness
Post-herpetic Neuralgia (PHN)	Prevention of PHN	88.2% vaccine effectiveness for prevention of PHN	85.6% vaccine effectiveness for prevention of PHN	• 30 days post vaccination up to 1 year: ARR = 0.0381%, NNT = 2,625 (1 case of PHN prevented for every 2,625 vaccinations) • 3 to 4 years post vaccination: ARR = 0.037%, NNT = 2,703 (1 case of PHN prevented for every 2,703 vaccinations)
Herpes Zoster Ophthalmicus (HZO)	Prevention of HZO	75.5% vaccine effectiveness for prevention of HZO	71.2% vaccine effectiveness for prevention of HZO	• 30 days post vaccination up to 1 year: ARR = 0.0349%, NNT = 2,865 (1 case of HZO prevented for every 2,865 vaccinations) • 3 to 4 years post vaccination: ARR = 0.0329%, NNT = 3,038 (1 case of HZO prevented for every 3,038 vaccinations)

Vaccine Safety

- Shingrix®[5] commonly reported adverse reactions
  - 49% Myalgia
  - 46% Fatigue
  - 40% Headache
  - 30% Shivering
  - 24% Fever
  - 17% GI symptoms—nausea, vomiting, diarrhea, abdominal pain, etc.

Serious Adverse Events

- Guillain-Barré Syndrome - GBS (FDA requires notice of GBS risk under Warnings and Precautions section of vaccine package insert)
- Autoimmune blistering skin disorders
- Exacerbation of rheumatoid arthritis
- Inflammatory bowel disorders
- Alopecia (hair loss)

Vaccine Safety Summary

Vaccine Safety	Details
Shingrix® Commonly Reported Adverse Reactions	
• Myalgia	49% of patients
• Fatigue	46% of patients
• Headache	40% of patients
• Shivering	30% of patients
• Fever	24% of patients
• GI symptoms (nausea, vomiting, diarrhea, abdominal pain, etc.)	17% of patients
Shingrix® Reported Serious Adverse Events	
• Guillain-Barré Syndrome (GBS)	FDA requires notice of GBS risk under Warnings and Precautions section of vaccine package insert
• Autoimmune blistering skin disorders	Rare
• Exacerbation of rheumatoid arthritis	Rare
• Inflammatory bowel disorders	Rare
• Alopecia (hair loss)	Rare

Conclusion

The combination of low effectiveness as measured by ARR and NNT with an exceptionally high-risk profile indicates benefits of Shingrix® do not outweigh the risks in healthy persons over fifty years of age. Antiviral therapy is available and can reduce duration of shingles episodes and severity of symptoms for those who develop herpes zoster.

Chapter Summary

Section	Key Points
Introduction	• Shingrix vaccine is recommended for adults ≥50 to prevent herpes zoster (shingles) and complications. • Chapter evaluates efficacy and safety, questioning benefits vs. risks for healthy older adults.
Shingles	• Caused by varicella-zoster virus (VZV), dormant after chickenpox, reactivating as shingles. • Symptoms: Painful rash (2–4 weeks), tingling, fever, potential postherpetic neuralgia (PHN). • Contagious via blisters (causes chickenpox in unexposed). • Risk factors: Age (>50), weakened immunity; complications include PHN, vision loss. • Treatment: Antivirals (e.g., acyclovir) and pain management.
Approved Shingles Vaccine	• CDC recommends Shingrix® (recombinant zoster vaccine, RZV) for ≥50 or immunocompromised ≥19. • Uses recombinant DNA to produce VZV antigen for immune response without causing disease.
Shingrix® Dosage	• Two doses recommended for eligible adults to prevent shingles and PHN.
Vaccine Effectiveness	• Shingles Prevention: Claimed 91% effective (Relative Risk Reduction, RRR); Actual 0.38% (Absolute Risk Reduction, ARR), NNT = 263. • PHN Prevention: Claimed 85% effective (RRR); Actual 0.36% (ARR), NNT = 277. • RRR from trials overstates benefit; ARR/NNT reflect low real-world impact.
Vaccine Safety	• Common Reactions: Myalgia (49%), fatigue (46%), headache (40%), shivering (30%), fever (24%), GI issues (17%). • Serious Adverse Events: Guillain-Barré Syndrome (GBS), autoimmune skin disorders, rheumatoid arthritis exacerbation, inflammatory bowel issues, alopecia. • FDA notes GBS risk in package insert.
Conclusion	• Low effectiveness (ARR, NNT) and high-risk profile suggest Shingrix® benefits do not outweigh risks for healthy ≥50 adults. • Antiviral therapy offers viable alternative to reduce shingles duration/severity.

CHAPTER 8

Pneumococcal Vaccines: Marginal Effectiveness with Significant Risks for Seniors

Pneumococcal vaccines are recommended for older adults to prevent serious infections like community-acquired pneumonia. This chapter evaluates their effectiveness and safety, highlighting concerns about limited clinical efficacy and significant adverse events.

The annual revenue for pneumococcal vaccines in the United States for 2024 is estimated at $8.49 billion, dominated by Pfizer's Prevnar 20®. This figure is expected to grow to $12.19 billion by 2030, with a compound annual growth rate (CAGR) of 6.21 percent from 2024 to 2030, driven by increasing demand for conjugate vaccines (PCVs) like Vaxneuvance, Prevnar 20, and CAPVAXIVE, which target a broader range of serotypes and offer higher efficacy compared to the polysaccharide vaccine (PPSV23, Pneumovax23). The suffix number in the vaccine name indicates the number of S. pneumoniae serotypes it covers, over one hundred of which have been identified.

Pneumococcal Infections

Pneumococcal infections, caused by *Streptococcus pneumoniae* (*S. pneumoniae*), pose a significant threat to seniors, particularly those over sixty-five. This bacterium can lead to serious conditions like pneumonia (lung infection), bacteremia (blood infection), and meningitis (infection of the lining of the brain and spinal cord), with older adults at higher risk due to weakened immune systems and chronic conditions.

Infection can lead to severe illness, hospitalization, and death. Common symptoms in the elderly may be subtle, such as confusion or low alertness, complicating early diagnosis. The CDC recommends pneumococcal vaccines (PCV20, PCV21, or PPSV23) for adults sixty-five and older to reduce risk. Additional prevention includes managing chronic conditions and avoiding long-term care facilities where infection rates are higher. Prompt treatment with antibiotics is crucial for bacterial cases.

Pneumonia

Pneumonia represents about 95 percent of serious *S. pneumoniae* conditions and can lead to bacteremia and meningitis. Pneumonia acquired in the community, known as Community-Acquired Pneumonia (CAP), is the most common form. Other types are Hospital-Acquired Pneumonia (HAP) and Nursing Home-Acquired Pneumonia (NHAP). HAP is less likely to be due to *S. pneumoniae* and more likely attributable to Staphylococcal or other bacterial infections whereas NHAP is still predominantly due to *S. pneumoniae*.

The CDC recommends the following pneumococcal vaccines for adults fifty years and older, or for adults nineteen to forty-nine with certain risk factors including diabetes, smoking history, sickle cell disease, immunocompromising conditions, and chronic illnesses. The number after each vaccine represents the number of serotypes or strains of the pneumococcal bacteria addressed by the vaccine.

There are two forms of pneumococcal vaccines, conjugated and unconjugated polysaccharides. First, polysaccharide is a complex sugar molecule derived from the outer capsule or shell of the bacteria. It serves as the antigen in all of the pneumococcal vaccines.

The difference is whether the polysaccharide is conjugated, that is, attached to a carrier protein or is unconjugated/ unattached. This attachment to a carrier protein serves to stimulate a different form of response from the immune system than the unconjugated polysaccharide, potentially resulting in stronger, more durable immunity. In addition, the conjugated vaccine reduces the likelihood of becoming an asymptomatic carrier of the bacteria in the nasopharynx.

Pneumococcal Vaccines

Vaccine Type	Specific Vaccine	Manufacturer	Approval Year (US)
Pneumococcal Conjugate Vaccines (PCVs)	PCV15—Vaxneuvance™	Merck & Co., Inc.	2021
	PCV20—Prevnar 20®	Pfizer	2021
	PCV21—CAPVAXIVE™	Merck & Co., Inc.	2024
Pneumococcal (unconjugated) Polysaccharide Vaccine	PPSV23—Pneumovax23®	Merck & Co., Inc.	1983 (updated)

Vaccine Effectiveness

Vaccine effectiveness of pneumococcal conjugate and polysaccharide vaccines is difficult to determine from existing studies. Vaxneuvance™, Prevnar20®, and CAPVAXIVE™ have not performed randomized, controlled clinical trials (RCTs) to establish effectiveness. Research demonstrating effectiveness has primarily focused on antibody studies. These investigations demonstrate "non-inferiority" (no worse than) in comparison with antibody responses to the various vaccine strains covered by previous versions of the vaccines. In other words, the assurance of vaccine effectiveness offered by the manufacturers is that the vaccine is no worse than earlier vaccines.

Prevnar13® - Foundation for most pneumococcal vaccines

Prevnar13®, approved in 2010, established the clinical basis for future pneumococcal conjugate vaccines. It is the only conjugate pneumococcal vaccine to undergo a randomized, placebo-controlled, clinical trial with a disease prevention endpoint (pneumonia). Multi-strain, conjugate vaccines released since Prevnar13® were approved based on antibody responses, not disease prevention studies. Consequently, all the successor pneumococcal vaccines rely on this vaccine to help support claims of clinical effectiveness.

The Prevnar13® study was conducted on nearly eighty-five thousand individuals aged sixty-five and older in the Netherlands to assess the effectiveness against pneumococcal infections, including community-acquired pneumonia (CAP).[1] Prevnar13® vaccine efficacy was reported to be just 46 percent. There was no difference in mortality between Prevnar13® and placebo.

Prevnar13® Clinical Trial Results

Metric	Value	Description
Claimed Vaccine Effectiveness Against CAP	46%	The vaccine is claimed to reduce the risk of CAP by 46% compared to placebo, based on clinical trial data.
Absolute Risk Reduction (ARR)	0.1%	The actual reduction in risk of CAP per 100 vaccinated individuals
Number Needed to Treat (NNT)	1000	For every 1000 people vaccinated, 1 person benefits by avoiding CAP, indicating a high NNT and relatively low individual benefit despite the claimed effectiveness.

Since Prevnar13® was released, evidence shows non-vaccine serotypes are increasing, which could reduce some benefits of the multi-strain vaccines.[2]

In summary, the clinical foundation for multi-strain, conjugate vaccines is a product released 15 years ago that had mediocre results at best, even using the manufacturers' RRR analysis. The more meaningful ARR analysis shows vaccine benefit approaching zero.

CAPVAXIVE™

The most recently released conjugate vaccine for adults is CAPVAXIVE™. Despite the absence of a number, the vaccine covers twenty-one serotypes. CAPVAXIVE™ shares coverage of fourteen serotypes with Pneumovax23®, adding seven emerging strains in what would seem to be an endless chase of new serotypes. However, CAPVAXIVE™ uses a different antigen that is said to elicit a stronger and longer-lasting immune response, particularly in adults.[3]

But does it? As with every pneumococcal vaccine since Prevnar13®, key clinical trials for CAPVAXIVE™ were restricted to antibody studies. As observed with previous vaccines, the trials established non-inferiority compared with previous vaccines' antibody studies (meaning no worse than previous vaccines) for most strains and some increased antibody response for other strains. It is worth emphasizing that antibody levels do not correlate with clinical effectiveness at preventing community-acquired pneumonia, yet these vaccines are promoted by the medical community as providing protection against CAP.

Pneumovax23®

Pneumovax23®, the sole approved unconjugated vaccine, claims effectiveness based on clinical trials. However, the package insert does not provide any data or references to support their conclusions. Merck claims 57 percent overall effectiveness for the vaccine's twenty-three pneumococcal strains for all ages, and 75 percent effectiveness in persons aged sixty-five years of age and older, based on CDC's pneumococcal surveillance system.[4] It is not possible to verify these claims or to subject the clinical trials data to more relevant ARR analysis without access to the primary data.

Vaccine Safety

Vaccine safety assessments may be constrained in several ways. First, comparators are typically other vaccines, or other vaccine ingredients minus the antigens, and not placebos. This reframes the assessment and diminishes safety signals which may appear in both groups. Vaccine studies also tend to report solicited adverse events, meaning they don't record all events but only those they list. Manufacturers may also limit the time period for review of adverse events to a few days or weeks after vaccination, missing longer-term safety signals such as heart, liver, or immune system effects.

Only post-marketing studies, required of the manufacturer by the FDA after vaccine approval, provide the most candid assessments of vaccine safety. These results are found in Section 6 of the package insert, titled "Adverse Reactions," which is read by few doctors and virtually no patients.

Two striking examples of pneumococcal vaccine adverse events follow.

Adverse Reaction	Percentage (%)
Muscle Pain	66%
Fatigue	43%
Headache	39%
Arthralgia	13%

Prevnar20® Commonly reported adverse reactions in individuals 60 years and older[5]

Pneumovax23® Serious Adverse Events[6]

Infrequent Serious Adverse Events*
Angina
Heart Failure
Ulcerative Colitis
Tremor
Depression
Stroke
Pancreatitis
Heart Attack
Guillain-Barré Syndrome
Death

*A serious adverse event is a harmful, potentially life-threatening reaction to a drug or vaccine requiring medical intervention.

It is evident from reported common and serious adverse events that pneumococcal vaccines carry a material degree of risk which is rarely discussed with patients.

Conclusion

Pneumococcal vaccines for the prevention of community-acquired pneumonia in healthy adults fifty years of age and older have marginal effectiveness, a high rate of common, moderately severe side effects, and a long list of less common serious adverse events. The foundation for newly released pneumococcal vaccines rests weak clinical results from a vaccine approved 15 years ago. None of the vaccines claim clinical effectiveness for the serotypes of pneumococcal bacteria not covered by the vaccines. At most, only twenty-three pneumococcal strains out of over one hundred are accounted for. Pneumococcal bacteria will continue to evolve and backfill around covered strains, requiring ever greater serotype coverage. Clinical studies that demonstrate vaccine effectiveness are limited and largely depend on comparative antibody studies. Antibody studies do not necessarily correlate with clinical effectiveness.

Chapter Summary

Section	Key Points
Introduction	• Pneumococcal vaccines target serious infections (e.g., pneumonia) in seniors; chapter assesses efficacy and safety. • 2024 US revenue: $8.49B (Pfizer's Prevnar 20® dominant), projected to reach $12.19B by 2030 (6.21% annual growth rate).
Pneumococcal Infections	• Caused by Streptococcus pneumoniae, risks seniors (>65) with pneumonia, bacteremia, meningitis. • Subtle symptoms (e.g., confusion) complicate diagnosis; CDC recommends PCV20, PCV21, or PPSV23. • Prevention includes managing chronic conditions; antibiotics treat bacterial cases.
Pneumonia	• 95% of serious S. pneumoniae cases; Community-Acquired Pneumonia (CAP) most common. • Hospital-Acquired (HAP) and Nursing Home-Acquired (NHAP) differ; NHAP still S. pneumoniae-dominant.
Pneumococcal Vaccines	• Conjugate Vaccines (PCVs): PCV15 (Vaxneuvance™, 2021), PCV20 (Prevnar 20®, 2021), PCV21 (CAPVAXIVE™, 2024) by Merck/Pfizer. • Polysaccharide Vaccine: PPSV23 (Pneumovax23®, 1983) by Merck. • Conjugation to carrier proteins enhances immunity, reduces asymptomatic carriage.
Vaccine Effectiveness	• No RCTs for PCV15, PCV20, CAPVAXIVE™; rely on antibody non-inferiority vs. prior vaccines. • Prevnar13® (2010): 46% efficacy against CAP, 0.1% ARR, NNT = 1,000 (no mortality difference). • CAPVAXIVE™: Covers 21 serotypes, claims stronger response via antibody studies (no clinical data). • Pneumovax23®: Claims 57% overall, 75% (>65) effectiveness (unverifiable, no ARR data).

Section	Key Points
Vaccine Safety	• Assessments limited by non-placebo comparators, solicited events, short review periods. • Prevnar20®: Muscle pain (66%), fatigue (43%), headache (39%), arthralgia (13%). • Pneumovax23®: Serious events include angina, heart failure, stroke, GBS, death. • Post-marketing data (Section 6) reveals risks rarely discussed.
Conclusion	• Marginal effectiveness (high NNT, no mortality benefit) with frequent side effects and serious risks. • Relies on weak Prevnar13® data; covers only 23/100+ serotypes, with evolving bacterial resistance. • Antibody studies lack clinical correlation; benefits questionable for healthy seniors ≥50.

CHAPTER 9

Respiratory Syncytial Virus (RSV): Still Searching for Evidence of Benefit

Respiratory syncytial virus (RSV) infection is a viral illness caused by RSV, a common respiratory virus. It typically presents as a mild cold-like illness with symptoms such as runny nose, cough, sore throat, fever, and fatigue. In most healthy adults, RSV is self-limiting and resolves within one to two weeks without specific treatment.

However, in older adults, those with weakened immune systems, or individuals with underlying conditions (e.g., heart or lung disease), RSV can lead to more severe complications, such as:

- Bronchiolitis: Inflammation of the small airways.
- Pneumonia: Infection of the lungs.
- Worsening chronic conditions such as COPD, congestive heart failure, or asthma.

Severe cases may require hospitalization, especially in adults over sixty-five or those with comorbidities. RSV is highly contagious, spreading through respiratory droplets or contact with contaminated surfaces. Older adults living in long-term care facilities have a higher incidence of the infection than the general population.

Below are estimates for the frequency of illness, serious disease, hospitalization, and mortality in this population, based on recent data (2022–2025) from sources such as the CDC, WHO, and peer-reviewed studies.

Clinical Burden of RSV

Category	Definition	Estimates	Relevance for 65+
Frequency of Illness	Symptomatic RSV infections, typically acute respiratory infections with cold-like symptoms (e.g., rhinorrhea, cough, fever).	• Incidence Rate: 0.6% for 65+ each year • Annual Cases: 890,000–1.7M in US • Underreporting: RSV in 5.5% of outpatient ARIs	Older adults (esp. 75+, Long Term Care Facilities (LTCF) residents more susceptible due to weaker immune systems; 17% of cases in LTCFs.
Serious Disease	Severe RSV causing lower respiratory tract infections (LRTIs) such as pneumonia, bronchiolitis, or exacerbations of chronic conditions (e.g., COPD, CHF).	• Prevalence: 57.8% of hospitalized 60+ have pneumonia • Complications: 19.4–25.6% have exacerbated chronic conditions; 14–22% have cardiovascular issues. • Proportion: 10–15% of 65+ cases progress to severe LRTIs.	More common in 75+ (54% of hospitalizations), LTCF residents (17.2%), and those with comorbidities (e.g., COPD, CHF).
Hospitalization	RSV-associated hospitalizations due to severe LRTIs, pneumonia, or exacerbated comorbidities.	• Annual Hospitalizations: 60,000–160,000 in US • Rate: 0.2% for 65+; 2.24% for 75–84. • ICU: 17.0% of hospitalized 60+.	Risk 10x higher for 75+ vs. 65–74; elevated in COPD, CHF, LTCF residents; 26.9% of 60+ in ICU
Mortality	RSV-associated in-hospital deaths or deaths within 60 days post-admission.	• Annual Deaths: 6,000–10,000 in US • Hospital Case Fatality Rate: 4.7% US • Risk Factors: Cancer treatment, age >75, LTCF residence	Significant in 75+, comorbidities (COPD, CHF), LTCFs; RSV mortality comparable to or exceeds influenza's (8% vs. 7%)

Note: Data is specific to adults 65+ unless noted.[1]

Approved RSV Vaccines

CDC recommends one of three vaccines for adults seventy-five years and older and for adults sixty years and older who are at increased risk of severe RSV infection—one dose and not given annually.[2]

Vaccine	Manufacturer	Approval Year
Abrysvo®	Pfizer	2023
Arexvy®	GSK	2023
mRESVIA®	Moderna—mRNA vaccine	2024

Vaccine Effectiveness

Abrysvo®
Significant discrepancy in vaccine effectiveness exists between manufacturer-reported calculation based on Relative Risk Reduction and the method used to measure drug effectiveness known as Absolute Risk Reduction. In this instance, 84 percent versus 1.5 percent vaccine effectiveness.

Category	Details
Product Claim	84% effectiveness (measured by Relative Risk Reduction—RRR) for the prevention of lower respiratory tract infection (LRTI)[3]
Actual Effectiveness	• No significant effect on prevention of hospitalization or severe illness • Effectiveness measured by Absolute Risk Reduction (ARR) is approximately 1.5% (ARR: the amount the vaccine reduces an individual's risk of a LRTI) • Number Needed to Treat = NNT 67* * NNT 67 means 67 adults need to be vaccinated for one person to avoid a LRTI. Few benefit, but all vaccinated assume potential vaccine risks • Subsequent analysis found an NNT 250** ** Kaiser Permanente of Southern California follow-up study for vaccine prevention of hospitalization or ED visit for pneumonia[4]

Arexvy®
Significant discrepancy in vaccine effectiveness exists between manufacturer-reported results based on a statistical method known as Relative Risk Reduction (RRR) and the technique often used to measure drug effectiveness, known as Absolute Risk Reduction (ARR). Pharmaceutical companies prefer to report results using RRR because it can heavily favor vaccine efficacy results in large clinical trials. In this instance, Arexvy® RRR produced 82 percent efficacy versus 0.2 percent vaccine effectiveness using the ARR calculation.

From a patient perspective, ARR presents a more realistic result because it reveals how much a vaccine reduces an individual's chances of getting a deep respiratory infection from RSV. In this example, a reduction in risk of only 0.2

percent from getting an RSV pneumonia makes a much less compelling case for the vaccine than the headline number of 82 percent.

Category	Details
Product Claim	82% effective by Relative Risk Reduction (RRR) for lower respiratory tract infection (LRTI)[5]
Actual Effectiveness	• No significant effect on prevention of hospitalization or severe illness • Absolute Risk Reduction (ARR) is 0.2% • NNT 500: Just one in 500 vaccinated people will avoid a LRTI

mRESVIA®

Significant discrepancy in vaccine effectiveness exists between manufacturer-reported calculation based on Relative Risk Reduction and the method used to measure drug effectiveness known as Absolute Risk Reduction. In this instance, 62.5 percent to 78 percent versus 0.6 percent vaccine effectiveness.

There is a massive difference in vaccine effectiveness between manufacturer-reported Relative Risk Reduction calculations and the Absolute Risk Reduction method used to measure drug effectiveness.

Category	Details
Claim	62.5% to 78% effective by Relative Risk Reduction (RRR) for lower respiratory tract infection (LRTI)[6]
Actual Effectiveness	• No significant effect on prevention of hospitalization or severe illness • Absolute Risk Reduction (ARR) is 0.6% • NNT 333: Just one in 333 vaccinated people will avoid a LRTI

Summary of RSV Vaccine Effectiveness

Vaccine	Claimed Effectiveness to Prevent LRTI (RRR)	Absolute Risk Reduction (ARR)	Effectiveness on Hospitalization or Severe Illness	Number Needed to Treat (NNT) for 1 Person to Benefit*
Abrysvo®	84%	1.5%	No significant effect on hospitalization or severe illness	67—250
Arexvy®	82%	0.2%	No significant effect on hospitalization or severe illness	500
mRESVIA®	62.5%–78%	0.6%	No significant effect on hospitalization or severe illness	333

* All vaccinated assume vaccine risks but as few as 1 in 500 benefit.

Vaccine Safety

RSV vaccines first received approval in 2023. Consequently, there are no long-term studies that evaluate vaccine safety.

In early 2025, the US Food and Drug Administration (FDA) announced the RSV vaccines marketed as Abrysvo® by Pfizer and Arexvy® by GSK will now require a warning about the risk of Guillain-Barré syndrome (GBS), a form of severe and potentially life-threatening paralysis occurring within forty-two days of the RSV shot. Moderna's mResvia, the only other FDA-approved RSV vaccine, has no such disclaimer.[7]

Abrysvo®

- Commonly reported adverse reactions[8]

Symptom	Percentage
Fatigue	16%
Headache	13%
Myalgia	10%
Arthralgia	8%
Diarrhea	6%

- Serious Adverse Events
  - Abrysvo® approved for use in older adults in May 2023
  - Data from post-release marketing studies tracking serious adverse events are still in process[9]
- Autoimmune neurological disorders already detected include:
  - Guillain-Barré Syndrome (GBS)
  - Miller Fisher Syndrome (related to GBS)
  - Motor-sensory axonal polyneuropathy (systemic injury to nerve cells, nerve fibers (axons) and protective nerve coverings)

Arexvy®

- Commonly reported adverse reactions[10]

Symptom	Percentage
Fatigue	34%
Myalgia	29%
Headache	27%
Arthralgia	18.1%

- Serious Adverse Events
  - FDA approval 2023 - Data from post-release marketing studies tracking serious adverse events are still in process
  - Reports from initial Study groups identified atrial fibrillation and some deaths

mResvia®

- Commonly reported adverse reactions

Symptom	Percentage
Fatigue	31%
Headache	27%
Myalgia	25%
Arthralgia	22%
Underarm swelling or tenderness	15%
Chills	11%

- Serious Adverse Events
  - Post-marketing studies limited by recent FDA approval in 2024
  - 8% incidence of serious adverse events during clinical trials
  - mRNA vaccines in general lack long-term safety testing and assume rapid degradation of mRNA in the body, inability of the mRNA or DNA plasmid contaminants to enter the cell nucleus, and there is no incorporation of DNA contaminants into the cellular DNA. There is considerable research that disputes these assumptions. See Chapter 5, COVID-19 mRNA Vaccines: Alarming Safety Signals and Regulatory Failures

RSV Vaccine Adverse Reactions

Vaccine	Commonly Reported Adverse Reactions	Serious Adverse Events
Abrysvo®	• Fatigue: 16% • Headache: 13% • Myalgia: 10% • Arthralgia: 8% • Diarrhea: 6%	• Approved May 2023 • Post-marketing studies ongoing • Autoimmune neurological disorders detected: Guillain-Barré Syndrome (GBS), Miller Fisher Syndrome, Motor-sensory axonal polyneuropathy

(continued . . .)

Vaccine	Commonly Reported Adverse Reactions	Serious Adverse Events
Arexvy®	• Fatigue: 34% • Myalgia: 29% • Headache: 27% • Arthralgia: 18.1%	• Approved 2023 • Post-marketing studies ongoing • Initial study reports: atrial fibrillation, some deaths
mResvia®	• Fatigue: 31% • Headache: 27% • Myalgia: 25% • Arthralgia: 22% • Underarm swelling/ tenderness: 15% • Chills: 11%	• Approved 2024 • Limited post-marketing data • 8% incidence of serious adverse events in clinical trials

Conclusion

RSV vaccines have shown minimal impact on lower respiratory tract infections without preventing serious illness or hospitalization. Their recent approval means long-term safety studies are still pending. The high incidence of systemic effects, potential neurological complications, and lack of sufficient post-marketing studies indicate that the benefits may not outweigh the risks for older adults. The CDC's Advisory Committee on Immunization Practices (ACIP) should reconsider their broad recommendation for older adults based on the recently reported increased risk of GBS. Additionally, the high incidence (one in twelve) of serious adverse events for the mRNA RSV vaccine recommends withdrawal pending separate long-term safety studies.

Chapter Summary

Section	Key Points
Introduction	• RSV causes mild, self-limiting cold-like illness in healthy adults (1–2 weeks); severe in older adults (≥65), immunocompromised, or those with comorbidities. • Complications include bronchiolitis, pneumonia, worsened chronic conditions; hospitalization risk rises with age/comorbidities.
Clinical Burden of RSV	• Frequency of Illness: 0.6% incidence in 65+, 890K–1.7M US cases/year, 5.5% of outpatient ARIs, 17% in Long Term Care Facilities (LTCFs). • Serious Disease: 57.8% of hospitalized 60+ have pneumonia, 10–15% of 65+ cases severe, 54% in 75+. • Hospitalization: 60K–160K US cases/year, 0.2% in 65+, 2.24% in 75–84, 17% ICU. • Mortality: 6K–10K US deaths/year, 4.7% hospital fatality, high in 75+, LTCFs, comorbidities (e.g., COPD, CHF).

Section	Key Points
Approved RSV Vaccines	• CDC recommends Abrysvo® (Pfizer, 2023), Arexvy® (GSK, 2023), mRESVIA® (Moderna, 2024) for ≥75 or at-risk 60+; single dose, not annual.
Vaccine Effectiveness	• Abrysvo®: Claimed 84% (RRR) vs. 1.5% (ARR), NNT 67–250, no significant hospitalization/severe illness prevention. • Arexvy®: Claimed 82% (RRR) vs. 0.2% (ARR), NNT 500, no significant hospitalization/severe illness prevention. • mRESVIA®: Claimed 62.5–78% (RRR) vs. 0.6% (ARR), NNT 333, no significant hospitalization/severe illness prevention. • RRR overstates benefit; ARR/NNT show minimal real-world impact.
Vaccine Safety	• Approved 2023–2024; no long-term data. • Abrysvo®: Fatigue (16%), headache (13%), myalgia (10%), GBS warning (2025), autoimmune neurological disorders. • Arexvy®: Fatigue (34%), myalgia (29%), atrial fibrillation, deaths reported. • mRESVIA®: Fatigue (31%), myalgia (25%), 8% serious adverse events, concerns over mRNA safety assumptions (see Chapter 5). • FDA added GBS warning for Abrysvo®/Arexvy®.
Conclusion	• Minimal impact on LRTI, no prevention of serious illness/hospitalization. • High systemic effects, neurological risks, and limited post-marketing data suggest risks outweigh benefits. • ACIP should reconsider recommendations; mRESVIA® (1 in 12 serious events) should be withdrawn pending long-term safety studies.

CHAPTER 10

Tetanus

Pro tip: When asked about getting a tetanus shot in the ER, ask if the shot prevents the wound from developing dangerous tetanus neurotoxin. It doesn't. Development of neutralizing antibodies from the vaccine takes 7–14 days, while the neurotoxin can develop within a few days if tetanus bacteria are present.

Tetanus, caused by the bacterium *Clostridium tetani*, is a severe and potentially fatal disease characterized by muscle spasms and rigidity, commonly known as "lockjaw." The disease is caused by tetanus toxin, produced by bacterium in wounds. The toxin inhibits neurotransmitter release, resulting in severe muscle contractions.[1]

Despite its rarity in developed countries, tetanus remains a significant global health concern, particularly in agrarian regions with regular exposure to cattle, horses and other farm animal manures which may harbor the bacteria.

Tetanus vaccine does not prevent infection. Rather, the vaccine uses a toxoid, which is an inactivated form of the tetanus toxin, to stimulate production of antibodies to neutralize tetanus toxin.[2]

This chapter examines the tetanus vaccine's mechanism, effectiveness, and associated concerns, including ingredients, adverse events, and the critical timing of its protective effect in emergency settings, alongside historical data on tetanus cases and deaths in the United States since 1960.

Tetanus Toxoid Vaccines

There is no such thing as a single vaccine tetanus "shot." The vaccine is always administered in combination with diphtheria (Td) or diphtheria and pertussis (DTaP or Tdap). Diphtheria is no longer endemic (circulating) in the US. Healthy adults are not at risk of serious pertussis infection. The T component of the vaccine targets the tetanus toxin rather than the bacterium. An upper-case D or P in the vaccine description indicates a higher dose than lower case d or p. The addition of diphtheria to the tetanus vaccine offers no additional benefit while incurring all its risks.

Below is a table summarizing the key tetanus toxoid-containing vaccines available in the United States (adult vaccines in shaded area):[3]

Vaccine Name	Aluminum Content	Formaldehyde Content	Other Ingredients	Target Population
Infanrix (DTaP)	500 mcg aluminum hydroxide (mcg = micrograms)	≤ 100 mcg	≤ 100 mcg Polysorbate 80 (TWEEN 80*)	Infants and children up to 7 years
DAPTACEL (DTaP)	1.5 mg aluminum phosphate (333 mcg aluminum)	≤ 5 mcg	< 50 ng residual glutaraldehyde, 3.3 mg 2-phenoxyethanol	Infants and children up to 7 years
Adacel (Tdap)	1.5 mg aluminum phosphate (333 mcg aluminum)	≤ 5 mcg	< 50 ng residual glutaraldehyde, 3.3 mg 2-phenoxyethanol	Adults and children aged 7 and up
Boostrix (Tdap)	300 mcg aluminum hydroxide	≤ 100 mcg	≤ 100 mcg Polysorbate 80 (TWEEN 80*)	Adults and children aged 7 and up
TDVAX (Td)	≤ 530 mcg aluminum	< 100 mcg	Trace thimerosal (≤ 0.3 mcg mercury/dose)	Adults and children aged 7 and up
TENIVAC (Td)	1.5 mg aluminum phosphate (330 mcg aluminum)	≤ 5.0 mcg	None listed	Adults and children aged 7 and up

Note: These vaccines contain adjuvants like aluminum, a known neurotoxin, to enhance immune response, preservatives like formaldehyde, and other components such as polysorbate 80 and 2-phenoxyethanol, which can have systemic effects, including neurological, renal, hepatic, and hematological toxicity.[4]

*The presence of polysorbate 80 and glutaraldehyde in vaccines, such as those for tetanus, has raised questions about their safety, particularly regarding allergic reactions and long-term effects on gut health, liver, and kidney toxicity.[5]

Side Effects of Tetanus-Containing Vaccines

While the tetanus vaccine is generally considered safe, it is not without potential side effects. The following table outlines common and more serious adverse events associated with these vaccines:[6]

Side Effect	Frequency	Description
Injection-site pain, redness, swelling	25–85%	Local reaction, typically resolving within days
Fever, fatigue	< 10%	Systemic symptoms
Anaphylaxis	1.6 per one million doses	Severe allergic reaction, requiring immediate medical attention (underreporting likely)
Guillain-Barré Syndrome (GBS)	Not quantified	Institute of Medicine report found evidence for a causal relationship of GBS with vaccination.[7] History of GBS a possible contraindication to vaccination.[8]
Brachial plexus neuropathy	5–10 per one million doses	Rare neurological complication
Deaths reported to VAERS	3,209 (as of recent data)	Includes all tetanus-containing vaccines (significant underreporting likely)
Anaphylaxis in milk-allergic individuals	Not quantified, but documented	Risk due to cow's milk protein in vaccine formulation

The presence of aluminum, formaldehyde, and cow's milk protein in these vaccines has been linked to anaphylaxis, particularly in individuals with known allergies. The Vaccine Adverse Events Reporting System (VAERS) data identifies significant adverse events, though underreporting is acknowledged.[9]

Mechanism and Effectiveness

The tetanus vaccine operates as an anti-toxin, stimulating the immune system to produce antibodies against the toxin produced by *Clostridium tetani*. Unlike most vaccines that target live pathogens, the tetanus toxoid is inactivated by formaldehyde, preserving its immunogenic properties while eliminating its toxicity.[10] This allows the body to generate antibodies that neutralize the toxin before it can bind to nerve cells, preventing the severe muscle spasms and rigidity associated with tetanus.

There are no placebo-controlled trials or long-term safety studies for the tetanus vaccines. Clinical effectiveness is determined by the capacity of the vaccine to produce neutralizing antibodies. The presence of antibodies does not necessarily correlate with clinical effectiveness.

A complete series consists of three doses for adults or four for children under seven years. Booster doses every ten years are recommended to maintain immunity, although a 2016 study suggested that protection may last up to thirty years, challenging the current schedule.[11]

The World Health Organization (WHO) does not recommend routine adult booster vaccination for tetanus and diphtheria after completion of the childhood vaccination series. A recent study that reviewed over eleven billion person-years of incidence data revealed no benefit associated with performing adult booster vaccinations against tetanus or diphtheria.[12]

Timing of Onset and Emergency Room Administration

A critical aspect of the tetanus vaccine's utility is its timing of onset, particularly in emergency settings where a contaminated wound poses an immediate risk. The tetanus vaccine does not provide immediate protection against tetanus toxin formation due to the delay in immune response. For individuals who have not been previously vaccinated or are under-vaccinated (fewer than three doses), the vaccine requires seven to fourteen days to generate a measurable immune response, with full protective antibody levels typically achieved after completing a three-dose primary series over several months.[13] This timeline is too slow to counteract the rapid onset of tetanus toxin production, which can occur within two to fourteen days post-exposure, depending on the wound's severity and contamination level.

In the emergency room (ER), where a tetanus-prone wound is treated, the vaccine's role is primarily preventive for future exposures rather than immediate protection against tetanus spores. Deep penetrating wounds contaminated by dirt or manure from farms, feed lots and stables environments and crush injuries are considered at higher risk. Thorough wound care, including cleaning and debridement, is a priority, as it removes *Clostridium tetani* spores and reduces the likelihood of toxin production.[14]

For unvaccinated or under-vaccinated individuals with high-risk wounds, in addition to thorough wound care, treatment may include both intravenous tetanus immune globulin (TIG) and a tetanus toxoid vaccine (e.g., Td or Tdap). TIG provides immediate passive immunity by supplying pre-formed antibodies via intravenous administration that neutralize unbound tetanus toxin, bridging the gap until the vaccine-induced immunity develops.[15]

Annual Tetanus Cases and Deaths in the United States Since 1960

The decline in tetanus cases and deaths in the US since 1960 is considered by the CDC the successful result of vaccination efforts. The following table provides the annual number of tetanus cases and deaths reported in the United States from 1960 to 2024, based on available data:[16]

Year	Number of Cases	Number of Deaths
1960	525	181
1970	146	47
1980	98	21
1990	64	10
2000	41	5
2010	26	3
2020	6	1 (underreported due to COVID pandemic)
2021	16	2
2022	28	3
2023	24	2 (Preliminary)
2024	22	2 (Preliminary)

This data illustrates a dramatic reduction in both tetanus cases and deaths since 1960, from 525 cases and 181 deaths in 1960 to an average of about 30 cases and 2.5 deaths per year since the 2000s. The decline is attributed to widespread vaccination but the counterargument emphasizes the role of non-vaccination factors.[17]

Impact of Improved Wound Care and Fewer Farm Workers

The decline in tetanus cases and deaths may not be solely attributable to vaccination but also to improved wound care practices and a reduction in the number of farm workers, who are at higher risk due to occupational exposure to *Clostridium tetani* spores in soil and manure. This perspective suggests that advancements in medical and public health practices, such as improved sanitation, better hygiene, antiseptic techniques, and prompt wound management, have significantly reduced the incidence of tetanus. For instance, the introduction of antibiotics and improved surgical debridement techniques have decreased the likelihood of *Clostridium tetani* proliferation in wounds, even before the toxin can be produced.[18]

Additionally, the shift in the US workforce away from agriculture, particularly since the mid-twentieth century, has reduced the population at risk. In 1960, approximately 8.3 percent of the US workforce was employed in agriculture, compared to about 1.3 percent in 2020.[19] This decline in farm workers, coupled with urbanization and changes in lifestyle, has decreased exposure to tetanus-prone environments. Historical data shows that tetanus cases were disproportionately higher among rural populations and farm workers, who were more likely to sustain contaminated wounds. As these groups diminished, so did the overall incidence of tetanus, irrespective of vaccination rates.[20]

Proponents of this counterargument also point to the timing of the decline in tetanus cases, which began before widespread vaccination was achieved. For example, between 1947 and 1960, tetanus cases dropped from around 580 to 525, and deaths declined from 460 to 181 during a period when vaccination coverage was still expanding but not yet universal or uniform. Furthermore, the decline in cases persisted during this period despite highly variable vaccine coverage across the states, supporting the idea that non-vaccination factors are significant.[21]

Ingredients and Adverse Events

The tetanus vaccines contain ingredients that have raised concerns, including aluminum (330–530 mcg per dose), formaldehyde (≤5–100 mcg), and cow's milk protein, which poses a risk of anaphylaxis in allergic individuals. VAERS data reports 3,209 deaths associated with these vaccines, though underreporting is acknowledged.[22] The use of Tdap in pregnancy, despite inadequate safety studies and concerns about miscarriage exclusion in research, adds complexity to its application (see Chapter 11: Vaccines and Pregnancy).[23] Financial motivations behind vaccination recommendations, as well as historical and ongoing debates about necessity and safety, suggest a need for transparent, evidence-based policy.[24]

Conclusion

The tetanus vaccine remains a cornerstone of public health, attributed to reducing tetanus incidence and mortality through its anti-toxin mechanism. However, the timing of its protective effect, particularly in emergency settings, underscores the importance of proper wound care and TIG for immediate intervention in contaminated wounds, as the vaccine alone cannot prevent toxin formation within the critical early days post-exposure. The decline in US tetanus cases and deaths since 1960 probably reflects the combined impact of vaccination, improved wound care, and a reduction in the number of farm workers, challenging the notion that vaccines alone are responsible. The WHO and retrospective studies do not support booster vaccination every ten years. Ongoing concerns about ingredients, adverse events, and the necessity of frequent boosters warrant careful consideration. The financial and policy motivations behind vaccination recommendations, coupled with the potential risks, highlight the need for informed consent and individualized risk assessment. Tetanus vaccine boosters for adults should no longer be required except for those at high risk and a single vaccine tetanus product uncombined with other vaccines such as diphtheria or pertussis should be made available.

CHAPTER 11

Vaccines and Pregnancy: Caveat Emptor

In pregnancy, as in healing, first do no harm; let caution guide every choice for mother and child.
—Adapted from the Hippocratic Oath (ca. 400 BCE)

The exposure of unborn children to maternal vaccination during pregnancy is often overlooked in discussions about vaccines. During this developmental stage, fetuses are sensitive to immune system stimulants and vaccine ingredients. There is limited discourse on the potential risks of fetal exposure to vaccination during pregnancy, with a greater focus on the benefits for mothers, infants, and society.

Therefore, we analyzed the potential risks and benefits associated with vaccines administered during pregnancy.

Both the CDC and the American College of Obstetrics and Gynecologists (ACOG) recommend that pregnant women receive several vaccines to protect themselves and their unborn children. These include influenza, Tdap, RSV, and COVID-19 vaccines, all of which the CDC asserts are safe for pregnant women and their fetuses.

However, none of these vaccines are approved by the FDA specifically for use during pregnancy, meaning they have not been tested in this population through FDA-authorized clinical trials demonstrating safety and efficacy. The term "approved" indicates that the vaccine has undergone such clinical trials and met predetermined safety and clinical outcome measures.

In 2019, ICAN (Informed Consent Action Network) asked for a copy of each report from the FDA of clinical trials that were used to support the safety of vaccines during pregnancy. The federal regulatory agency was required by law to supply this information under the FOIA (Freedom of Information Act).

When the FDA failed to respond to the request, a lawsuit followed that suggested they had never licensed a vaccine to be used for pregnant women. The FDA responded to this inquiry stating, "We have no records responsive to your requests." This means the FDA had NO RECORDS of any clinical trial that a vaccine was ever tested on pregnant women to ensure its safety.[1]

As a result, the package inserts for these vaccines do not indicate approval for use during pregnancy. It is noteworthy that both the FDA and CDC presume that if vaccines are approved for adult use, they must be safe for pregnant women and their babies.

This chapter will review claims of safety and efficacy for each of the vaccines recommended during pregnancy, present updated information from clinical studies, and discuss the controversy around recently appointed HHS Secretary Kennedy's recommendation to remove the COVID-19 vaccine from CDC's recommended vaccines during pregnancy schedule.

CDC Recommended Vaccines (v) by Trimester

Vaccine	1st Trimester	2nd Trimester	3rd Trimester
Tdap	X	X	✓
Flu (inactivated)	✓	✓	✓
COVID-19*	✓	✓	✓
RSV	X	X	✓

* Health Secretary Robert F. Kennedy Jr. announced in May 2025 that the CDC would no longer recommend COVID-19 vaccination during pregnancy. However, as of publication, the CDC still explicitly recommends vaccination:

"Everyone, including women who are pregnant, should stay up to date with their COVID-19 vaccines, including getting an updated vaccine when it's time to get one."[2]

Secretary Kennedy's position is strongly disputed by the American College of Obstetricians and Gynecologists.[3]

With the premise that a baby gets disease protection from their mother during pregnancy, the CDC states that vaccination allows the mother to pass protective antibodies on to their unborn child. The CDC also assures that these four vaccines are safe for pregnant women and their babies.

All mothers and parents-to-be deserve access to better information than CDC assurances so they can make informed decisions about vaccinations during pregnancy. The following sections discusses each of the four recommended vaccines. After detailed analysis of the evidence, the data support rejection of any of the listed vaccines for pregnant women in good health.

PART I: INFLUENZA VACCINES

Are Flu Vaccines Safe for Pregnant Women?

A 2021 *JAMA* study claimed that vaccines posed no risk for pregnant women.[4] The study authors posed the question: "Is seasonal influenza vaccination in pregnancy associated with adverse childhood outcomes?" Their answer was that there was no *significant* association with adverse childhood outcomes among vaccinated offspring. However, according to Brian Hooker, PhD, the researchers got it wrong.

In the study, out of a cohort of 28,255 children born in Nova Scotia, 36 percent were exposed to the influenza vaccine during gestation. The researchers followed the children's health for an average of 3.6 years and concluded there were no associated adverse outcomes reported (including asthma, upper and lower respiratory infections, gastrointestinal infections, abnormal tissue growths, and hearing or vision loss).

The study failed to consider several factors when drawing this conclusion. The researchers relied only on ER and hospital data and ignored outpatient records that recorded higher rates of GI and lower respiratory infection. Authors also claimed no difference in outcomes between the vaccinated and unvaccinated, despite ear infections occurring at a higher rate in the vaccinated group. Lastly, the all-cause injuries (meaning injuries from any cause) in the control diagnosis group showed significantly higher numbers in the maternally vaccinated children as compared to the unvaccinated.

Study: Spontaneous Abortions

In 2017, the CDC published a seismic study that directly linked spontaneous abortions in women to flu vaccines.[5] In a review of data from the 2010–2011 and 2011–2012 flu seasons, women who were vaccinated with the inactivated influenza virus had twice the chance of a spontaneous abortion within twenty-eight days of receiving the inoculation. The most alarming statistic to come out of this study was that in women who received the H1N1 vaccine, there was a 7.7 times greater incidence of a miscarriage in the twenty-eight days following the shot. Despite the threat to the unborn child, the CDC still recommended all flu vaccines that contain the H1N1 strain for use during pregnancy.

Other Related Risks: Inflammation, Autism, and Diabetes

Inflammation

Beyond the risk of a spontaneous abortion, there are several other increased risks from taking the flu vaccine. A primary impetus for giving the vaccine is to promote an immune response, which, starting with the innate (quick response) immune system, is by definition inflammatory.

Inflammation is a natural part of the body's defense system, helping the body to recognize harmful foreign substances (such as a virus) and begin healing and recovery.[6]

In utero, inflammation can also have serious consequences, including an increased risk for psychiatric disorders and autism. The trivalent influenza virus vaccination has been shown in studies to cause a measurable inflammatory response which is associated with adverse health outcomes for the mother and child.[7]

Autism

One of these adverse health outcomes is autism. A 2014 study reinforces the notion that inflammation during pregnancy, regardless of whether from vaccines, is associated with autism.[8] Alan Brown, MD, and his colleagues found that of the 1.2 million pregnant women studied, elevated CRP levels were associated with a 43 percent greater risk of having a child with autism. Keep in mind that CRP, or C-reactive protein, is the same marker of inflammation that increases after flu vaccination.

A 2021 study also concluded that maternal immune activation plays a significant role in the pathogenesis of autism. Inflammation and associated cellular stress have been reported in the brain tissues of individuals diagnosed with autism spectrum disorder. The study authors stated the inflammatory processes (like those that happen after flu vaccination) cause a "self-perpetuating vicious cycle that leads to abnormalities in brain development and behavior."[9]

Gestational Diabetes and Eclampsia

Gestational diabetes, pre-eclampsia, and eclampsia are serious conditions that can develop during pregnancy, posing a risk for both mother and baby. Pre-eclampsia is characterized by high blood pressure, edema or water retention, and protein in the urine. This condition can cause a number of problems for a pregnant woman and baby, including low birth weight and risk of hemorrhage during childbirth. It can also lead to eclampsia (dangerous seizures that are life-threatening). Gestational diabetes is a form of diabetes that only develops in pregnancy and is associated with elevated blood sugar levels that can lead to an increased risk for C-section, pre-eclampsia, and depression.

Another study published in the *British Medical Journal* reported that the influenza vaccine increased the risk for gestational diabetes and life-threatening eclampsia.[10] In 2014, Giuseppe Traversa and colleagues assessed maternal, fetal, and neonatal outcomes of women given the influenza A/H1N1 vaccine. The outcomes of over eighty-six thousand pregnancies revealed that vaccinated women had significantly higher rates of gestational diabetes and eclampsia.

Birth Defects

In a 2016 study, Chambers et al. found a moderately elevated risk for birth defects among children born to mothers who received one flu vaccine during the 2010–2014 flu seasons.[11] A closer look at the study revealed that exposure to the vaccine during the first trimester was associated with nearly twice as many major birth defects than among the unexposed babies (5.7 percent vs. 3.0 percent).

Marginally Effective Outcomes

Each year, influenza vaccines are formulated based on strains identified months in advance based on global flu surveillance. All flu vaccines in the US are "quadrivalent," meaning they are based on four different flu viruses (two influenza A viruses and two influenza B viruses). The CDC *guesses* which strains will predominate in the US in the coming flu season based on what strains are in circulation in the southern hemisphere six months in advance.

Every year, flu vaccine effectiveness (VE) rarely rises above 50 percent. For example, the 2021–2022 flu season saw a 16 percent VE rate, the 2022–2023 flu season reports a 23 percent VE rate against hospitalizations for adults aged eighteen to sixty-four years, and a study from the Cleveland Clinic found that vaccinated employees were 27 percent more likely to become infected than their unvaccinated peers.[12, 13, 14]

When adverse effects from flu vaccines are considered, the risk-to-benefit ratio does not support vaccination for most people. Yet, the push is on each year to get everyone vaccinated.

Do Repeat Vaccinations Increase the Risk of Infection?

At least two studies suggest repeated influenza vaccinations increase the risk of influenza infection. The latest was co-authored by the CDC's own investigators who found that there was an 11 percent increase in the rate of infection following vaccination for certain strains.[15] The authors speculated about factors that may have contributed to increased risk of infection following repeat vaccination but concluded they "cannot fully explain the increased infection risk in repeat vaccinees compared with non-repeat vaccinees."[16]

This investigation follows a similar report from 2015 when Canadian researchers found those vaccinated during the prior flu season had a 15 percent increased risk of infection compared to the unvaccinated.[17]

Observation of negative effectiveness has driven some Canadian public health officials to reconsider universal flu vaccine programs. Ontario's former chief medical officer, once a proponent of universal programs stated,

"We should . . . do a very careful rethink of where we are. There's enough new evidence that we should all be troubled enough by . . . our policies. There are more and more unanswered questions about how effective a universal program really is."[18]

Perhaps the experts in the CDC US Flu Vaccine Effectiveness Network should consider these sentiments and acknowledge that, much like with the COVID-19 mRNA vaccines, repeat immunization against the same virus has been shown to diminish an effective antibody immune response.[19]

Profitable Vaccine with Recurring Revenue

While not very effective for most people, influenza vaccines generate steady cash flow year in and year out. Flu vaccines are a big profit center, generating nearly $7 billion in annual revenue and expected to grow to $10 billion by 2028.[20] There has never been a successful vaccine developed to prevent any of the common respiratory viruses that afflict humans, despite billions of research dollars. They simply mutate too quickly. Yet, they remain widely embraced by the public and the medical community. Look for increased promotion of combination influenza-COVID-19 vaccines in an effort to reverse declining sales of the unpopular COVID-19 vaccines.

Conclusion: Influenza Vaccine

On balance, a risk-benefit assessment of influenza vaccination supports removal from recommended vaccines for pregnant or women who are in good health. The influenza vaccine was never tested on pregnant women prior to approval. The testing since approval in support of its use is equivocal to contradictory. Several studies point strongly to the potential for harm to babies, including an increased risk for autism, gestational diabetes, eclampsia, asthma, and gastrointestinal disorders. Lastly, the flu vaccine is marginally effective (as low as 13 percent to minus 26 percent) even if it were safe.[21] It is unclear whether influenza vaccination in high-risk pregnancies or for mothers with chronic illnesses offers any better risk-benefit profile than for healthy mothers-to-be.

Part I Summary

Topic	Summary
FDA's Lack of Safety Data	• In 2019, ICAN requested FDA clinical trial reports on vaccine safety in pregnancy via FOIA. The FDA's failure to respond led to a lawsuit, revealing no records of clinical trials testing vaccine safety in pregnant women. • The FDA's response, "We have no records responsive to your requests," indicates no vaccine has been licensed specifically for use in pregnant women based on pregnancy-specific safety trials.
Safety Claims and Critiques	• A 2021 JAMA study claimed no adverse childhood outcomes (e.g., asthma, infections, sensory loss) from maternal influenza vaccination, based on 28,255 children (36% exposed in utero) followed for 3.6 years. • Brian Hooker, PhD, critiqued the study for ignoring outpatient records showing higher GI and lower respiratory infections, higher ear infection rates in vaccinated children, and significantly more all-cause injuries in vaccinated vs. unvaccinated children.
Spontaneous Abortion Risks	• A 2017 CDC study linked flu vaccines to a doubled risk of spontaneous abortion within 28 days of vaccination during the 2010–11 and 2011–12 flu seasons. • Women receiving the H1N1-containing vaccine had a 7.7 times higher miscarriage risk within 28 days, yet the CDC continues to recommend H1N1-containing flu vaccines for pregnant women.
Other Health Risks	• Inflammation: Flu vaccines induce an inflammatory immune response, which in utero increases risks of psychiatric disorders and autism. A 2014 study linked elevated CRP (inflammation marker post-vaccination) to a 43% higher autism risk. • Autism: A 2021 study confirmed maternal immune activation (e.g., post-vaccination inflammation) contributes to autism via a "self-perpetuating vicious cycle" affecting brain development. • Gestational Diabetes & Eclampsia: A 2014 BMJ study of 86,000+ pregnancies found vaccinated women had higher rates of gestational diabetes and life-threatening eclampsia, increasing risks of low birth weight, hemorrhage, and C-sections. • These conditions pose significant risks to maternal and fetal health, including neonatal complications and maternal mortality.

(continued . . .)

Topic	Summary
Birth Defects	• A 2016 study by Chambers et al. reported a moderately elevated risk of birth defects in children of mothers vaccinated during the 2010–14 flu seasons. • First-trimester exposure was linked to nearly twice as many major birth defects (5.7% vs. 3.0% in unexposed), highlighting early pregnancy risks.
Vaccine Effectiveness	• Flu vaccines are quadrivalent, targeting four strains predicted from global surveillance. • Effectiveness (VE) is often low: 16% in 2021–22 and 23% against hospitalizations in 2022–23 for adults 18–64, and a negative 27% in 2024–2025. • The low VE (rarely above 50%) and potential adverse effects result in a poor risk-to-benefit ratio for most people, including pregnant women.
Risks of Repeat Vaccination	• Two studies suggest repeat flu vaccinations increase infection risk: a CDC study found an 11% higher infection rate for certain strains, and a 2015 Canadian study reported a 15% increased risk in previously vaccinated individuals. • Negative effectiveness has prompted some Canadian officials to question universal flu vaccine programs, citing unanswered questions about efficacy.
Profit Motives	• Flu vaccines generate ~$7 billion annually, projected to reach $10 billion by 2028, despite low effectiveness and rapid viral mutation. • Efforts to combine flu and COVID-19 vaccines aim to boost declining COVID-19 vaccine sales, highlighting commercial interests over public health benefits.
Conclusion	• The risk-benefit assessment strongly advises against flu vaccination in healthy pregnant women due to untested safety in pregnancy, equivocal or contradictory post-approval studies, and risks of spontaneous abortion, autism, gestational diabetes, eclampsia, asthma, GI disorders, and birth defects. • With marginal effectiveness (13% to negative 26%), the flu vaccine offers limited benefits, even for high-risk pregnancies or mothers with chronic illnesses. • The recommendation for flu vaccination in pregnant women should be withdrawn based on the lack of robust safety and efficacy data.

PART II: COVID-19 VACCINES

The CDC recommends:

> "Everyone ages 6 months and older is recommended to get the updated COVID-19 vaccine, including if you are pregnant, breastfeeding a baby, trying to get pregnant now, or might become pregnant in the future."

The CDC further states that the COVID vaccines are safe and effective:

> "Evidence shows that COVID-19 vaccination before and during pregnancy is safe and effective and suggests that the benefits of vaccination outweigh any known or potential risks."[22]

Notably, CDC's position is strongly endorsed by the American College of Obstetricians and Gynecologists.

ACOG's Vaccine Advocacy

The American College of Obstetricians and Gynecologists (ACOG) claims to be the "premier professional membership organization for obstetricians and gynecologists," counting over sixty thousand members across North and South America. Most obstetricians belong to ACOG and are influenced by its policies.

ACOG strongly disputes HHS Secretary Kennedy's position on changing the CDC's recommendation from comprehensive recommendation to conditional subject to shared clinical decision-making with a woman's practitioner. They state:

> "The American College of Obstetricians and Gynecologists (ACOG) strongly recommends that all pregnant individuals receive the updated 2024–2025 COVID-19 vaccine, citing extensive evidence of its safety and effectiveness in protecting both pregnant women and their newborns from severe COVID-19 complications, including hospitalization, preterm birth, and stillbirth. ACOG opposes the US Department of Health and Human Services' (HHS) May 2025 decision to stop recommending routine COVID-19 vaccination for healthy pregnant women, arguing it undermines vaccine confidence and ignores robust data showing reduced maternal and fetal risks. Pregnant women are encouraged to discuss vaccination with their healthcare providers, but documentation of such discussions is not required."[23]

ACOG is not without potential conflicts of interest in its advocacy position. Confidential documents obtained under a Freedom of Information Act (FOIA) request reveal the potential for undue influence between the federal Health and Human Services (HHS), the Center for Disease Control (CDC), and the American College of Obstetricians and Gynecologists (ACOG).[24]

On April 1, 2021, the Department of Health and Human Services formally introduced the COVID-19 Community Corps, a membership organization formed to promote vaccines to as many people as possible.[25] HHS had a war chest of over $16 billion in grant money to be awarded to non-government organizations (NGOs) to recruit what HHS refers to as "trusted community leaders."

In this campaign, HHS targeted 275 influential NGOs and health and medical organizations, including the AMA, American Academy of Pediatrics, and the ACOG. These organizations, influencers, and individuals could serve as "trusted messengers" to promote the COVID-19 vaccine.

HHS hoped that their vaccine promotion would penetrate even the most sacrosanct of relationships, that between a patient and her doctor. ACOG joined the Community Corps as a founding member, ultimately receiving millions in HHS/CDC grant money. As of 2022, ACOG received grants totaling over $11 million to promote COVID-19 injections.

As will be discussed below, compelling evidence disputes both the safety and effectiveness of COVID-19 vaccination during pregnancy. COVID-19 vaccines have not been shown to prevent severe disease from current variants and considerable risks to the fetus have been identified.

CDC Views Pregnancy as a Disease

As discussed in Chapter 5: COVID-19 Vaccines: Alarming Safety Signals and Regulatory Failures, CDC has implemented a new Regulatory Framework that establishes those considered to be high risk from COVID-19. Along with various chronic illnesses, cancer, and heart disease, CDC decided to include "Pregnancy and Recently Pregnant." In effect, pregnancy is considered a disease state and recently pregnant women, many of whom are breastfeeding, are considered prime candidates for COVID-19 vaccination. This decision completely ignores the established science of mRNA distribution across the placental membrane and in breast milk discussed below.

Maternal COVID Vaccination Fails to Protect Babies

The CDC, HHS, and the ACOG promote COVID-19 vaccines for pregnant women, promising protection for their unborn babies. In fact, the CDC directly states on their "Pregnant and Protected" website that "[w]omen who are vaccinated before or during pregnancy or while breastfeeding are protected from getting very sick; [they also] help protect their babies from serious illness caused by COVID-19."[26]

However, studies show that this statement lacks broad scientific support.

A close look at a study published in *JAMA Network Open* reveals that vaccination during pregnancy has unacceptably low vaccine effectiveness.[27] The study authors looked at a cohort of 7,292 infants aged six months or older to see if they were protected from COVID after vaccination. The results revealed that vaccination before or during pregnancy did not influence babies testing positive with Omicron-variant.

Further, Goh and colleagues from the *JAMA* study reported low estimated vaccine effectiveness of 15.4–26.2 percent, far below the typical threshold for vaccine approval of 50 percent. Based on this data, vaccine risks appear to outweigh potential benefits.

Pfizer and FDA Hid Data

It was revealed in April 2023 that Pfizer and the FDA knew in early 2021 that the modRNA vaccine caused severe fetal harm and posed risks to breastfed infants. The information was contained in documents released under court order, which would have otherwise been withheld from public view for seventy-five years.[28]

Among the documents released was one titled "Pregnancy and Lactation Cumulative Review" that summarized clinical trial data through February 2021. The information was brought to light by a team of clinicians, attorneys, statisticians, and other volunteers organized by the *Daily Clout* who combed through thousands of pages of released documents.[29] A copy of the original Pfizer report can be found at this reference.[30]

Clinical trials typically exclude pregnant and lactating women from participating due to the increased risk to developing fetus and child, a practice observed during the Pfizer studies.[31] However, many of the exposures occurred as a result of vaccination prior to or during the first trimester—before women knew they were pregnant or were to become pregnant.

What is revealed in their document is chilling. Of the 673 cases identified by Pfizer, 458 involved exposure during pregnancy; 54 percent of these reported adverse events. These include fifty-one cases of spontaneous abortion, six premature labor and delivery cases (including two newborn deaths), one case of newborn severe respiratory distress, and a case of fetal tachycardia with an irregular heart rate over 180 beats per minute that required early delivery and hospitalization.

Of 673 cases, 215 involved exposure of infants during breastfeeding. Of these 215 babies, 41 suffered a range of adverse events, including fever, rash, irritability, diarrhea, lethargy, vomiting, agitation, and facial paralysis.

Just three days after Pfizer signed off on their internal report, the CDC announced in a White House press briefing that they recommended pregnant people receive a COVID-19 vaccination.[32]

Evidence for Increased Risk for Spontaneous Abortion

Two early studies contended that mRNA vaccines were safe in pregnant women. Both were seriously flawed but are frequently cited as evidence for vaccine safety.

A *New England Journal of Medicine* study titled "Preliminary Findings of mRNA Covid-19 Vaccine Safety in Pregnant Persons" claims to demonstrate the safety of mRNA COVID-19 vaccine during pregnancy. However, researchers used a study design that artificially lowered the rate of spontaneous abortion and stillbirth, augmenting the limited data available on the safety of the vaccine.[33]

The study reported a rate of spontaneous abortion following vaccination no different than that found in the general population. However, a closer look at the data shows that over 80 percent of trial participants were women vaccinated in their third trimester—well after the highest risk for spontaneous abortion.[34] Had these women been excluded from the study, the rate of spontaneous abortion miscarriage rises significantly above the norm, resulting in a markedly different conclusion about vaccine safety.

Concerns raised by the *NEJM* study about the increased risk of miscarriage following COVID-19 vaccination are supported by findings from a 2023 study published in the *British Journal of Obstetrics and Gynaecology* (*BJOG*).[35] This article *also* purports to show that there was no increase in miscarriage following vaccination.

However, a look at the raw data from the *BJOG* study tells a very different story. Instead of no effect, the raw data reveal a near doubling of the rate of miscarriage in the vaccine group compared with the unvaccinated group. In order to arrive at the original conclusion, the study authors introduced an entirely new and irrelevant detail: the incidence of induced abortions.

Failed Pregnancies Surge after COVID-19 Vaccination in Israeli Women

A recently published study strongly contradicts the findings of *NEJM* and *BJOG* studies cited above. Led by Dr. Josh Guetzkow, the study discovered a 43 percent increase in fetal losses among women vaccinated with mRNA COVID-19 vaccines during weeks eight to thirteen of pregnancy.[36] The study was based on over two hundred thousand pregnancies recorded in Israeli health data, one of the first nations to implement widespread COVID "vaccination" and one of the earliest to comprehensively study potential adverse effects.

mRNA Dose 1 showed 43 percent more losses and mRNA dose 3 showed a 19 percent increase. Late losses after week 24 were higher (2.7 percent for dose 1, 1.8 percent for dose 3 vs. 1.1 percent overall). Conversely, flu vaccination showed five fewer losses per 100, indicating lower risk. The study mitigates healthy vaccinee bias—where healthier individuals are more likely to vaccinate—by comparing flu and COVID-19 vaccine outcomes, strengthening the evidence of mRNA vaccines' biological risk.

Vaccine	Gestational Weeks	Observed Fetal Loss Rate (per 100)	Expected Fetal Loss Rate (per 100)	Difference (per 100)	Stillbirths (After Week 24)
mRNA Dose 1	8–13	13	9	+3.9 (43% increase)	2.7% (145% increase)
mRNA Dose 3	8–13	12	10	+1.9 (19% increase)	1.8% (64% increase)
Influenza	8–13	-5 less than expected	Expected	-5	Not reported
Overall (All Women)	-	-	-	-	1.1%

Study of 1.3 Million Women Links COVID Vaccines to Pregnancy Risk

A peer-reviewed study published in the *International Journal of Risk & Safety in Medicine* revealed that women vaccinated against COVID-19 had a "substantially lower" rate of successful conceptions—pregnancies resulting in live births—compared to unvaccinated women.[37] The study, conducted by researchers from the Czech Republic, Denmark, and Sweden, analyzed data from 1.3 million women aged eighteen to thirty-nine in the Czech Republic from January 2021 to December 2023.

By June 2021, successful conception rates were notably lower for vaccinated women, a trend persisting into 2022, when unvaccinated women's rates were approximately 1.5 times higher. The lack of convergence in conception rates over time between the two groups suggests potential long-term impacts of vaccination on reproductive health.

The study highlights the need for further research, as clinical trials conducted prior to FDA approval did not assess the vaccines' effects on fertility, despite known impacts on menstrual characteristics. Most vaccinated women received Pfizer or Moderna vaccines.

Vaccine LNP and mRNA Spread to Placenta and Umbilical Cord Blood

The placenta, like the blood-brain barrier, has long protected fetuses and brains from multiple pathogens and toxic agents. Lipid nanoparticles or LNPs, have been cleverly designed to circumvent both. Multiple studies have established the uptake of mRNA-carrier, lipid nanoparticles (LNPs) in the placenta.[38, 39]

Placental uptake of LNPs suggests that mRNA will also likely transfer to the cord blood of fetuses. Pfizer and Moderna animal studies detected the presence of lipid nanoparticles containing COVID-19 mRNA in placental tissues and other fetal organs.[40]

A 2024 study published in the *American Journal of Obstetrics and Gynecology* assessed whether COVID-19 vaccine mRNA was present in the placenta and cord blood following maternal vaccination during pregnancy.[41] Researchers at NYU School of Medicine detected vaccine mRNA in two placentas tested as well as in the cord blood of one of the patients (cord blood was not tested in the second patient).

The study authors conclude:

> "Our findings suggest that the vaccine mRNA is not localized to the injection site and can spread systemically to the placenta and umbilical cord blood. The detection of the spike protein in the placental tissue indicates the bioactivity of the vaccine mRNA reaching the placenta.
>
> To our knowledge, these two cases demonstrate, for the first time, the ability of the COVID-19 vaccine mRNA to penetrate the fetal-placental barrier and reach the intrauterine environment."[42]

Fibrous Clots Found in Young Children of Vaccinated Mothers

> *"Prion-like amyloid fibrils were found in the blood of chronically ill children who had been exposed to Pfizer's mRNA injections in utero. . . . We are potentially looking at a generational health crisis"*[43]

Blood clotting abnormalities have been frequently reported post COVID-19 mRNA vaccination.[44, 45] This has raised concerns about the potential for prolonged biological activity of spike proteins following fetal exposure. Amyloid fibrils are misfolded proteins or peptides that form insoluble, fibrous structures in the blood.[46]

A recent report found the presence of amyloid fibrils in the blood of a chronically ill three-year-old child with documented fetal exposure to maternal mRNA-based COVID-19 vaccination.[47] The affected child was born without vital signs just one week after the mother received her second Pfizer dose. The child was successfully resuscitated at birth but suffers from multiple, ongoing health problems. The discovery of amyloid fibrils in the blood is consistent with reports of post-vaccination clotting abnormalities in vaccinated adults. [48, 49]

Preconception and Beyond

A 2023 study of preconception concluded that COVID-19 vaccination in either partner at any time before conception is not associated with an increased rate of miscarriage. To arrive at that conclusion, researchers asked couples trying to get pregnant if they had been vaccinated and how many times. Couples were then followed through subsequent pregnancies, comparing the rate of miscarriage between vaccinated and unvaccinated couples.

Everything seemed straightforward until researchers "adjusted" the data to form groups of similar risk for miscarriage. An independent analysis of the data reveals that the researchers excluded those most at risk of miscarriage from the vaccinated group of their analysis.[50] Without explanation, researchers "excluded 75 vaccinated women, most likely to miscarry, for each similarly situated unvaccinated woman."[51]

Another 2023 study published in *Journal of Medical Virology* revealed that newborn babies are 1.78 times more likely to contract COVID-19 during the first six months of life after maternal vaccination compared with unvaccinated mothers.[52] The study was a meta-analysis of thirty previous studies representing over eight hundred thousand pregnancies and undermines the argument that the vaccine protects neonates.

Elevated Risk of Myocardial Injuries in Women

A 2023 study titled "Sex-specific differences in myocardial injury incidence after COVID-19 mRNA-1273 booster vaccination" followed 777 health-care workers who had been vaccinated with a Moderna booster.[53] The authors reported a high incidence of myocardial injury markers three days after vaccination, especially in women. Twenty of twenty-two participants who experienced myocardial injuries were female. The study concluded that myocardial injury was more common than previously thought and occurred more frequently in women than men.

Pregnancy is accompanied by remarkable changes in the cardiovascular system.[54] These include increases in heart rate, cardiac output (the volume of blood pumped from the heart), fluid volume, and changes in blood pressure. For example, by the fifth week of pregnancy, the cardiac output increases to 50 percent above pre-pregnancy levels.[55]

All these factors combined place quite a stress on the woman's body which can uncover underlying cardiovascular disease.[56] In fact, the leading cause of maternal deaths (33 percent) is cardiovascular disease, with over 50 percent of these deaths occurring postpartum.[57]

Considering the female predominance of myocardial injury as noted in this study, pregnant women may be at elevated risk of injury and death from mRNA COVID-19 vaccine.

Conclusion: COVID-19

Federal agencies like the HHS and CDC, along with professional organizations such as the ACOG, remain in full support of vaccination prior to and during all trimesters of pregnancy. The evidence from multiple studies is equivocal at best, and some study designs resulted in misleading results, creating a false sense of COVID-19 safety during pregnancy and subsequent neonatal immunity. The new Regulatory Framework that includes Pregnancy and Recent Pregnancy as indications for vaccination are misguided. Based on the available evidence, the recommendation to vaccinate pregnant and recently pregnant women should be withdrawn.

Part II Summary

Topic	Summary
CDC Recommendations	• The CDC claims COVID-19 vaccines are "unlikely to pose risk" for pregnant people but acknowledges limited safety data. It includes "Pregnancy and Recently Pregnant" in its high-risk Regulatory Framework, treating pregnancy as a disease state alongside chronic illnesses. • The CDC recommends vaccination during pregnancy or breastfeeding to protect mothers and babies from severe COVID-19, despite evidence of mRNA crossing the placental barrier and appearing in breast milk. • Recommendations lack support from published, peer-reviewed, controlled clinical trials for safety and effectiveness in pregnancy.
ACOG's Vaccine Advocacy	• The American College of Obstetricians and Gynecologists (ACOG), with over 60,000 members, joined the HHS's COVID-19 Community Corps in April 2021 to promote vaccines. • FOIA documents reveal ACOG received over $11 million in HHS/CDC grants by 2022 to act as a "trusted messenger" for vaccine promotion, raising concerns about undue influence. • ACOG's advocacy targets the patient-doctor relationship, encouraging obstetricians to promote COVID-19 vaccination to pregnant women.

Topic	Summary
Vaccine Effectiveness	• A JAMA Network Open study of 7,292 infants showed maternal vaccination (before or during pregnancy) had low effectiveness (15.4–26.2%) against Omicron-variant infections in infants, far below the 50% threshold for vaccine approval. • The study found no significant protection for infants, contradicting CDC claims that maternal vaccination protects babies from serious COVID-19 illness.
Pfizer and FDA Data Suppression	• In April 2023, court-ordered documents revealed Pfizer and the FDA knew by February 2021 that the mRNA vaccine caused fetal harm, including 51 spontaneous abortions, 6 premature labors (2 newborn deaths), and other adverse events in 458 pregnancy exposures. • Among 215 breastfeeding cases, 41 infants experienced adverse events (e.g., fever, rash, irritability, facial paralysis) from vaccine exposure via breast milk. • Despite this, the CDC recommended vaccination for pregnant people three days after Pfizer's internal report, with data withheld from the public for 75 years until released by Daily Clout's efforts.
Spontaneous Abortion Risks	• A *New England Journal of Medicine* study claimed no increased spontaneous abortion risk post-vaccination, but over 80% of participants were vaccinated in the third trimester, after the highest miscarriage risk period, skewing results. • A 2023 BJOG study reported no miscarriage increase but manipulated data by including induced abortions. Raw data showed a near doubling of miscarriage rates in vaccinated vs. unvaccinated groups. • These studies suggest a significant increase in spontaneous abortion risk when data is not manipulated. • Israeli study shows 43% surge in fetal loss among women vaccinated early in pregnancy.
Lipid Nanoparticle (LNP) and mRNA Distribution	• Lipid nanoparticles (LNPs) in mRNA vaccines bypass the placental barrier, with studies detecting vaccine mRNA in placental tissues and umbilical cord blood. • A 2024 *American Journal of Obstetrics and Gynecology* study found vaccine mRNA in two placentas and one cord blood sample, confirming mRNA crosses the fetal-placental barrier, with bioactive spike protein detected in placental tissue.

(continued . . .)

Topic	Summary
Amyloid Fibrils and Clotting	• A 2025 report identified amyloid fibrils (misfolded proteins forming insoluble clots) in the blood of a chronically ill three-year-old born to a mother vaccinated with Pfizer's mRNA vaccine during pregnancy. • The child, born without vital signs a week after the mother's second dose, was resuscitated but has ongoing health issues, consistent with post-vaccination clotting abnormalities in adults. • Amyloid fibrils suggest prolonged spike protein activity, potentially causing a "generational health crisis."
Preconception and Neonatal Risks	• A 2023 preconception study claimed no increased miscarriage risk post-vaccination, but researchers excluded 75 high-risk vaccinated women per unvaccinated woman, skewing results. • A 2023 *Journal of Medical Virology* meta-analysis of 800,000+ pregnancies found newborns of vaccinated mothers were 1.78 times more likely to contract COVID-19 in the first 6 months, undermining claims of neonatal protection.
Myocardial Injury Risks	• A 2023 study in *European Journal of Heart Failure* reported myocardial injury markers in 20 of 22 health-care workers (all but two female) three days post-Moderna booster, indicating higher risk in women. • Pregnancy increases cardiac output by 50% by week 5, stressing the cardiovascular system. With cardiovascular disease causing 33% of maternal deaths (50% postpartum), mRNA vaccines may elevate injury and mortality risks in pregnant women.
Conclusion	• Federal agencies (HHS, CDC) and ACOG strongly support COVID-19 vaccination before and during pregnancy, despite equivocal or misleading study results that falsely suggest safety and neonatal immunity. • Evidence shows increased risks of spontaneous abortion, placental mRNA transfer, amyloid fibril-related clotting, neonatal COVID-19 infection, and myocardial injury, particularly in women. • The CDC's Regulatory Framework classifying pregnancy as a high-risk condition is misguided. Based on the evidence, recommendations for vaccinating pregnant and recently pregnant women should be withdrawn.

PART III: TDAP VACCINES

In 2012, the CDC began recommending the Tdap vaccine (tetanus toxoid, reduced diphtheria toxoid and acellular pertussis) for pregnant women during their third trimester. They currently recommend that the vaccine should be given during each pregnancy, stating that women can give their babies protection against pertussis (whooping cough) before they are born.[58, 59]

The FDA's original approval of the two Tdap brands (Boostrix and Adacel) in the mid-2000s was as a booster for teens and adults, and the product inserts state that Tdap should be given during pregnancy only "when benefit outweighs risk." At the time of the 2011 recommendation, no prelicensure studies of Tdap safety during pregnancy were available, so most of the (largely unpublished) data used to justify the recommendation came from post-licensure pregnancy surveillance studies conducted by conflicted vaccine manufacturers.

CDC Advocates for Tdap Vaccination During Third Trimester

According to the CDC, infants are most vulnerable to pertussis infection during their first six months as they build immunity from vaccination. Consequently, the CDC recommends mothers receive third trimester vaccination to protect the child during the first six months of life by the passive transfer of maternal antibodies. CDC claims vaccination during pregnancy prevents 78% of cases and 90% of hospitalizations in infants younger than two months.

The CDC's Tdap recommendation is consistent with the other three vaccines also promoted during pregnancy: RSV, influenza, and COVID-19. Common to all these recommendations is the absence of published, peer-reviewed, controlled clinical trials regarding vaccine safety and effectiveness during pregnancy.

Additionally, the CDC's claim of third-trimester vaccine Tdap effectiveness was not the result of a prospective clinical trial in pregnancy. Rather, the CDC's recommendation was based on reanalysis of four previous observational studies which used a non-US formulation.

Put plainly, the CDC extracted data from old retrospective, observational studies, then recombined the data and subjected it to various statistical analyses to arrive at their estimate of vaccine effectiveness using a vaccine not available in the US.

Weak Evidence for Safety and Effectiveness During Pregnancy

For one of two Tdap brands (Boostrix®), a single clinical trial of a few hundred pregnant women (341 in Tdap group, 346 placebo) was used to justify the safety of the vaccine during pregnancy.[60] The trial included no long-term safety data and was never published in a peer-reviewed journal.

Adacel®, a second brand of Tdap, cites a single reanalysis of retrospective data obtained from an unrelated study as the basis for estimating vaccine effectiveness.[61] The reanalysis was conducted on a total of 271 cases of which thirty-two were given Adacel during the third trimester. Again, there was no prospective, controlled, randomized trial cited as evidence of safety or effectiveness.

Suppression of Infant Immune Response to Pertussis

A study of immune responses of infants born to mothers who received Tdap during pregnancy found diminished antibody responses to pertussis antigens compared with infants whose mothers received placebo during pregnancy.[62] The clinical implications of this finding are unknown but certainly run contrary to the prevailing concept of a protective shield while an infant builds immunity.

Increased Risk for Congenital Birth Defects

Tdap vaccine is recommended in the third trimester only in pregnant women, presumably to protect the fetus from vaccine toxicity during the first two trimesters. This is a justifiable concern. A 2023 study published in peer-reviewed *Infectious Diseases and Therapy* reveals the potential for an elevated risk of congenital birth defects attributed to the vaccine.[63]

The study, titled "Investigating Tetanus, Diphtheria, Acellular Pertussis Vaccination During Pregnancy and Risk of Congenital Anomalies," analyzed the incidence of congenital birth defects among 16,350 and 16,088 live-born infants in Tdap-exposed and unexposed live-births. The authors concluded that in eight body systems (eye, ear/face/neck, respiratory, upper GI tract, genitals, kidneys, and musculoskeletal system), there was a 17–100 percent+ greater chance of congenital malformation after vaccination.

Despite the concerning correlation between congenital defects and vaccinations, the study authors conclude that the vaccine is safe for pregnant women.

Conclusion: Tdap

The 2 FDA-approved Tdap vaccines are Adacel® and Boostrix®. According to the manufacturer's package insert for each, safety and effectiveness have not been established in pregnant women.[64, 65] The available evidence suggests children exposed to Tdap during pregnancy may not have adequate protection against pertussis infection and may have a higher risk of congenital abnormalities. Fetal safety and efficacy have not been established and the recommendation to vaccinate pregnant women should be withdrawn.

Part III Summary

Topic	Summary
CDC Recommendations	• Since 2012, the CDC has recommended the Tdap vaccine (tetanus toxoid, reduced diphtheria toxoid, and acellular pertussis) for pregnant women during the third trimester of each pregnancy to protect infants from pertussis (whooping cough) via maternal antibody transfer. • The CDC claims Tdap vaccination during pregnancy prevents 78% of pertussis cases and 90% of hospitalizations in infants under 2 months, based on a reanalysis of four retrospective, observational studies using a non-US Tdap formulation, not prospective clinical trials. • The recommendation aligns with other vaccines (RSV, influenza, COVID-19) promoted during pregnancy, all lacking published, peer-reviewed, controlled clinical trials for safety and effectiveness in pregnant women.
Evidence for Safety and Effectiveness	• The FDA approved Tdap vaccines (Boostrix® and Adacel®) in the mid-2000s as boosters for teens and adults, with package inserts stating use in pregnancy only when benefits outweigh risks. • No prelicensure safety studies for Tdap in pregnancy were available in 2011; the CDC relied on unpublished post-licensure surveillance studies by manufacturers. • Boostrix®: Safety based on one unpublished clinical trial with 341 vaccinated and 346 placebo pregnant women, lacking long-term safety data. • Adacel®: Effectiveness estimated from a reanalysis of retrospective data from an unrelated study (271 cases, 32 vaccinated in third trimester), with no prospective, controlled, randomized trial.
Immune Response Suppression	• A study found infants born to mothers vaccinated with Tdap during pregnancy had reduced antibody responses to pertussis antigens compared to infants of placebo-receiving mothers. • The clinical implications are unclear but contradict the notion of Tdap providing a protective immune shield for infants building immunity.

(continued . . .)

Topic	Summary
Risk of Congenital Birth Defects	• A 2023 peer-reviewed study in *Infectious Diseases and Therapy* analyzed 16,350 Tdap-exposed and 16,088 unexposed live births, finding a 17–100%+ increased risk of congenital malformations in eight body systems (eye, ear/face/neck, respiratory, upper GI tract, genitals, kidneys, musculoskeletal) among Tdap-exposed infants. • Despite these findings, the study authors concluded the vaccine is safe for pregnant women. • Tdap is recommended only in the third trimester, likely to minimize fetal exposure to potential vaccine toxicity in earlier trimesters.
Conclusion	• The FDA-approved Tdap vaccines (Adacel® and Boostrix®) have not established safety or effectiveness in pregnant women, per their package inserts. • Evidence suggests infants exposed to Tdap in utero may have inadequate pertussis protection and an elevated risk of congenital abnormalities. • Due to insufficient fetal safety and efficacy data, the recommendation for Tdap vaccination in pregnant women should be withdrawn.

PART IV: RSV VACCINES

On September 22, 2023, the CDC's Advisory Committee on Immunization Practices recommended pregnant women between thirty-two and thirty-six weeks get vaccinated against the respiratory syncytial virus (RSV) with the recently FDA-approved Abrysvo®.[66] The CDC stated that all infants should be protected against RSV using Pfizer's Abrysvo®, either in utero or shortly after birth. Abrysvo's antigen component contains recombinant RSV preF A and RSV preF B, two genetically engineered copies of proteins on the virus's surface that enable the virus to enter host cells.

The CDC further noted that in clinical trials among pregnant women at twenty-four through twenty-six weeks, there were more preterm births observed among the RSV vaccine recipients than the unexposed. Other notable occurrences were a higher rate of pre-eclampsia, lower birth weight, and jaundice in the pregnant RSV-vaccinated women.[67] Despite these observations, the CDC promotes the vaccine during the last trimester of pregnancy.

What Is RSV?

According to the CDC, RSV (respiratory syncytial virus) is a common respiratory virus that usually causes mild, cold-like symptoms that last for between one to two weeks.[68] RSV is the most common cause of lower respiratory tract infections in young children and adults. For the vast majority of people, RSV infection is like a cold. Accordingly, true prevalence (frequency in the population) is relatively unknown as the only people who are tested for it are those who are severely ill or in the hospital.[69]

ACOG recommends that pregnant women receive a single dose of Abrysvo® between thirty-two weeks and thirty-six weeks plus six days of gestation during the RSV season, typically from September through January in most parts of the US.[70]

Was There Adequate Informed Consent During Clinical Trials?

Reported rising numbers of RSV infections and hospitalizations prompted major drug manufacturers to quickly develop vaccines.[71] In the drive to develop an RSV vaccine for pregnant women, two companies jumped on board: GlaxoSmithKline (GSK) and Pfizer. In early 2022, both were working on RSV-F protein vaccines to inoculate pregnant women to protect their babies.

Abruptly, GlaxoSmithKline halted their phase three trial upon observing a higher incidence of preterm deliveries in RSV-vaccinated pregnancies compared with the placebo group.[72] According to the FDA, the researchers recorded nearly a 40 percent increase in preterm births in the vaccine arm of the study.[73]

Pfizer continued with their trial but chose to withhold the GSK trial information from their pregnant study participants, which raised concerns over the thoroughness of informed consent.[74] Accordingly, the *BMJ* (*British Medical Journal*) investigated Pfizer's RSV vaccine clinical trial and the failure to share this information with the pregnant women.[75]

In their investigation, *BMJ* examined trial consent forms that stated the vaccine was "risk-free" for the baby. The *BMJ* also contacted governmental health authorities and trial investigators in the eighteen countries where trials were being conducted globally, asking if informed consent was provided. No one responded.

Preterm Births, Jaundice, Low Birth Weight, and Pre-eclampsia

Like the GSK clinical trial, more preterm births were observed among those vaccinated than those who received the placebo in Pfizer's Abrysvo® trial.

The Abrysvo® package insert states:

> "Although not statistically significant, in the full trial population more preterm births and hypertensive disorders of pregnancy (including pre-eclampsia) were observed in persons administered the vaccine rather than the placebo, and more infants whose mothers received the vaccine had low birthweight ≤5.5 lbs (≤2,500 g) and neonatal jaundice compared with infants whose mothers received the placebo."[76]

The lack of statistical significance should be taken with a grain of salt. The placebo comparison group as with most vaccine clinical trials was not an inert substance that would establish a fair baseline. Rather, the placebo contained all the same excipients (ingredients) as the vaccine except for the RSV antigens. According to the package insert, the vaccine contained:

> "[placebo] contains the following buffer ingredients: 0.11 mg tromethamine, 1.04 mg tromethamine hydrochloride, 11.3 mg sucrose, 22.5 mg mannitol, 0.08 mg polysorbate 80, and 1.1 mg sodium chloride per 0.5 mL [dose]."[77]

Nevertheless, CDC brushed off concerns about observed disorders of pregnancy. They only required the vaccine label the potential risk as a warning and approved the vaccine for use in pregnant women at thirty-two to thirty-six weeks, citing a need to avoid the potential risks associated with a preterm birth before thirty-two weeks.[78]

The World Health Organization and current studies, however, note that preterm births *less than thirty-seven weeks of age* are the leading cause of neonatal morbidity and mortality globally.[79, 80] Thus the restriction beginning at thirty-two weeks should not assure mothers about the potential effect of the vaccine on neonatal development and health.

The CDC reported that the Pfizer trial found infants born to vaccinated mothers were more likely to have a low birth weight and neonatal jaundice. Low birth weight babies are twenty times more likely to develop complications and die in comparison to normal weight babies.[81] Severe jaundice in newborns can cause brain damage, cerebral palsy, and hearing loss.[82]

Hypertension and pre-eclampsia occurred more frequently in vaccinated pregnant women than in those who were unvaccinated. Pre-eclampsia increases a woman's risk of organ damage to the kidneys, liver, and brain.[83] This hypertensive disorder can also increase the risk for developing life-threatening complications during birth, such as placenta separation and hemorrhage.[84]

Pre-eclampsia can progress to eclampsia, uncontrollable seizures that, when left untreated, can cause the death of both the mother and baby. Women who survive preeclampsia have reduced life expectancy and an increased risk of cardiovascular disease, diabetes, and stroke.[85] Babies born from preeclamptic pregnancies have increased risks of preterm births, perinatal death, and neurodevelopmental delay.[86]

Guillain-Barré Syndrome (GBS)

In January 2025, the FDA required safety labeling changes for two RSV vaccines—Pfizer's Abrysvo® and GSK's Arexvy®—to include a warning about an increased risk of GBS within 42 days of vaccination.[87] This decision was based on a post-marketing observational study, clinical trial data, and reports to the Vaccine Adverse Event Reporting System (VAERS). The study, which analyzed Medicare claims data from May 2023 to July 2024, suggested an elevated risk, though the evidence was not strong enough to confirm a definitive causal relationship.

The FDA has required and approved safety labeling changes to include a new warning about the risk of Guillain-Barré syndrome (GBS) in the Warnings and Precautions section of the prescribing information for both vaccines.

Conclusion: RSV

In 2023, the CDC recommended that all pregnant women vaccinate with Pfizer's Abrysvo® RSV-vaccine to protect their unborn babies from the common respiratory virus. In their Morbidity and Mortality Weekly Report, the CDC informed the public that the pregnant women who received the vaccine experienced higher rates of preterm births and preeclampsia.[88]

The report also stated that infants of vaccinated mothers had higher rates of jaundice and low birth weights. The ACIP (Advisory Committee on Immunization Practices) concluded that the benefits of the vaccine at thirty-two to thirty-six weeks' gestation outweighed these "potential" risks, and the FDA subsequently granted approval.

In early 2025 FDA required safety labeling changes for Pfizer's Abrysvo® to include a warning about an increased risk of GBS within forty-two days of vaccination.

The FDA should rescind its approval of Pfizer's Abrysvo® vaccine during pregnancy. At minimum, FDA should require a Black Box warning about the neonatal risks from use during pregnancy.

Part IV Summary

Topic	Summary
CDC Recommendations	• On September 22, 2023, the CDC's Advisory Committee on Immunization Practices (ACIP) recommended that pregnant women at 32–36 weeks gestation receive Pfizer's Abrysvo® RSV vaccine to protect infants in utero or post-birth. • The American College of Obstetricians and Gynecologists (ACOG) endorses a single dose of Abrysvo between 32 weeks and 36 weeks + 6 days during RSV season (September–January in most US regions). • Despite higher rates of preterm births, pre-eclampsia, low birth weight, and jaundice observed in clinical trials, the CDC promotes vaccination in the last trimester, citing benefits outweighing risks.
RSV Overview	• RSV is a common respiratory virus causing mild, cold-like symptoms lasting 1–2 weeks, per the CDC. • It is the leading cause of lower respiratory tract infections in young children and adults but is typically mild, resembling a cold. • True prevalence is unknown as testing is primarily conducted in severe or hospitalized cases.

Topic	Summary
Informed Consent Issues	• GlaxoSmithKline (GSK) halted its phase 3 RSV vaccine trial in early 2022 due to a ~40% increase in preterm births in the vaccine group compared to placebo, as reported by the FDA. • Pfizer continued its Abrysvo trial but did not disclose GSK's findings to participants, raising concerns about informed consent. • The BMJ investigated Pfizer's trial, noting consent forms claimed the vaccine was "risk-free" for babies. BMJ contacted health authorities and investigators in 18 countries, but none confirmed informed consent was adequately provided.
Observed Adverse Outcomes	• Preterm Births: Pfizer's trial showed more preterm births in the vaccine group than the placebo group, though not statistically significant. The placebo contained active excipients (e.g., tromethamine, sucrose, mannitol), not an inert substance, potentially skewing comparisons. • Low Birth Weight: Infants of vaccinated mothers had a higher incidence of low birth weight (≤5.5 lbs or ≤2,500 g), increasing complication and mortality risks by 20 times compared to normal-weight infants. • Jaundice: Neonatal jaundice was more frequent in infants of vaccinated mothers, with severe cases potentially causing brain damage, cerebral palsy, or hearing loss. • Pre-eclampsia/Hypertension: Vaccinated pregnant women had higher rates of hypertensive disorders, including pre-eclampsia, which increases risks of organ damage (kidneys, liver, brain), placenta separation, hemorrhage, and eclampsia (seizures). Pre-eclampsia survivors face reduced life expectancy and elevated risks of cardiovascular disease, diabetes, and stroke. Babies from preeclamptic pregnancies have increased risks of preterm birth, perinatal death, and neurodevelopmental delay.

Topic	Summary
Guillain-Barré Syndrome (GBS)	• In January 2025, the FDA required safety labeling changes for Pfizer's Abrysvo and GSK's Arexvy to include a warning about an increased risk of GBS within 42 days of vaccination. • The decision was based on a post-marketing observational study (Medicare claims data, May 2023–July 2024), clinical trial data, and Vaccine Adverse Event Reporting System (VAERS) reports, though evidence was not strong enough to confirm a definitive causal link. • - The GBS warning is included in the Warnings and Precautions section of the prescribing information for both vaccines.
Conclusion	• In 2023, the CDC recommended Abrysvo for pregnant women to protect infants from RSV, despite trial data showing increased risks of preterm births, pre-eclampsia, low birth weight, and jaundice. The ACIP concluded that benefits at 32–36 weeks gestation outweighed these risks, leading to FDA approval. • In 2025, the FDA added a GBS warning to Abrysvo's labeling. Given the observed adverse outcomes, particularly the serious risks to neonatal and maternal health, the FDA should rescind approval of Abrysvo for use during pregnancy or, at minimum, require a Black Box warning to highlight neonatal risks.

CHAPTER 12

Gardasil® and HPV— High Risk, Low Reward

On June 8, 2006, the FDA licensed the first HPV-vaccine, Gardasil® (Merck), to be used primarily for girls and women between the ages of nine and twenty-six.[1] Subsequently, the CDC recommended routine HPV vaccination at ages eleven to twelve years as the primary measure to protect children from "certain cancers later in life."[2] They also advise that, if children start their vaccine series on or after fifteen years of age, three doses should be given over six months. Further, the CDC recommends that females through the age of twenty-six and males through age twenty-one should have "catch-up vaccinations."[3]

Background

Human papillomavirus (HPV) is a common sexually transmitted disease (STD) that is known to be highly contagious.[4] Some types of HPV may increase the risk for developing certain types of cancer, especially cervical.[5] The CDC heavily promotes these vaccinations, stating that they protect people from getting infected with specific cancer-causing HPV-type strains.

HPV is characterized by warts or lesions that may develop into cancer. Currently, there are over six hundred strains of HPV, with twelve identified as "high-risk HPV" types.[6] Of these, two are found in most HPV-related cancers: HPV 16 and HPV 18.[7]

HPV and Cervical Cancer

The National Cancer Institute (NCI) states that "virtually all cervical cancer" is caused by the HPV virus.[8] NCI also affirms that, in most people, the immune system clears the infection (typically within a year or two) without causing cancer.[9]

The average age of HPV-related cancer diagnosis is between fifty and sixty-eight years.[10] Cervical cancer is the most common type of HPV-associated cancer, and it is usually diagnosed earlier than the others, at age fifty. Globally, the median age of cervical cancer diagnosis is fifty-three, and for those in whom the cancer proves fatal, the average age at death being fifty-nine.[11]

Type of Cancer	Average age of diagnosis
Cervical	50
Vaginal	68
Vulvar	67
Anal	63 (women), 61 (men)
Mouth/Throat	63 (women), 61 (men)

Average age (years) that HPV-associated cancer occurs in women and men, according to the CDC.[12]

CDC's HPV-Vaccine Campaign

HPV vaccine promotional campaigns target millions of preadolescent and adolescent children for whom the risk of developing cervical cancer is remote. School-age children at no risk of developing HPV-related cancers are being vaccinated with multiple doses during their primary years of sexual development. Some cancers, such as vaginal and vulvar, are typically diagnosed around age sixty-eight—a fifty-five-year gap between vaccination and the potential onset of cancer.

According to the National Cancer Institute, the rate of new cervical cancer cases is 7.7 per one hundred thousand women per year.[13] This means that in any given year, .008 percent of all women in the United States are diagnosed with cervical cancer. The low incidence stands in stark contrast to promotional messaging that vaccines are essential to curb an epidemic of HPV-related cancers.

The central message of the promotional campaigns is to protect yourself and protect others you care about from a cancer-causing infection. This is a compelling and emotional appeal, but it is a distortion of reality. The human immune system and regular Pap smears are generally all the protection needed to prevent cervical cancer except for those who suffer from a rare genetic predisposition to cancer or are immune suppressed.

Considering the unlikelihood of adolescents and teens developing cervical and other HPV-related cancers, one would think that HPV vaccine risks should be near zero for taking the shots. Unfortunately, this is not the case.

Vaccine Effectiveness

HPV vaccines have never been shown to prevent cancer. Based on a Relative Risk Reduction calculation, HPV vaccines are 98 percent to 100 percent effective at preventing precancerous changes to the most superficial layer of cervical cells, the epithelia, over a three-year period.[14] It should be noted that precancerous changes are not the same as cancer.

However, using clinical study data provided in the Gardasil®9 package insert, the Absolute Risk Reduction is roughly 1.5 percent.[15] In other words, a woman of average risk reduces her chances of precancerous changes by just 1.5 percent from vaccination. This means that out of one hundred vaccinated women, sixty-six need the full series of vaccinations to prevent one woman from getting precancerous changes to cervical epithelial cells (not cancer).

Even accepting the claim of 98 to 100 percent risk reduction numbers, it is not possible to correlate inhibition of precancerous changes in the cervical epithelium with cancer prevention due to two main factors.

First, the average lag time between precancerous cells and the diagnosis of cancer is over twenty years.[16] It is not possible to assess vaccine efficacy with respect to cancer prevention within a three-year time frame allotted for most studies.

Second, around 98 to 99 percent of precancerous conditions will resolve on their own.[17, 18] Most are the result of inflammation or infection. Around three million women have abnormal Pap tests each year, yet fewer than 1 percent will be diagnosed with cancer.[19] Moreover, cervical cancer is generally regarded as treatable and curable, particularly if diagnosed at an early stage.

Researchers Express Caution

In an editorial that accompanied the key HPV vaccine study cited above, editors wisely raised another issue perhaps more important than the clinical results. They stated,

> "We must also carefully monitor for unintended adverse consequences of vaccination. For example, when selective immunologic pressure is applied with vaccination, the potential exists for non-vaccine-related strains [of HPV] to emerge as important oncogenic serotypes."[20]

Their concerns were justified. HPV strains not covered by the vaccines are posing new cancer threats, as discussed below.

HPV-Vaccine Safety Examined

In the 2.5 years immediately following Gardasil® approval in 2006, over twelve thousand adverse events were reported to the FDA's Vaccine Adverse Event Reporting System (VAERS). Among these reports were 772 serious adverse events, including Guillain-Barré syndrome, motor neuron disease, and pancreatitis; there were also thirty-two deaths with an average age of eighteen.[21]

Since 2006, 136 million doses of HPV vaccine (and counting) have been given to children and young adults in the United States. In this period, three vaccines have been developed and licensed by the FDA:

- Gardasil® (stopped marketing in 2017)
- Cervarix (approved in 2009 and withdrawn from the market in 2016)
- Gardasil®9 (approved in 2014)

Gardasil®9, the only HPV vaccine currently approved for use in the US, protects against nine HPV types (strains), including 6, 11, 16, 18, 31, 33, 45, 52, and 58.[22]

The CDC assures the public that HPV vaccines "are very safe," with the benefits outweighing the potential risks of the vaccine.[23] They also report that each of the three vaccines that have been used in children and adults were extensively safety tested in clinical trials. The CDC asserts that in these trials, each "HPV vaccine was found to be safe and effective."[24]

Despite these assurances, HPV vaccination side effects are common and include headaches, nausea, dizziness, and fainting.[25, 26] Further, HPV vaccine has been shown to increase the risk for developing chronic immune, neurological, and pain disorders, among other serious adverse events.[27] Plausible associations exist between HPV vaccines and autoimmune disorders, premature ovarian failure, Guillain-Barré Syndrome, and postural orthostatic tachycardia syndrome (POTS).[28, 29]

Gardasil®9 has not been evaluated for the potential to cause carcinogenicity or genotoxicity (damage to genes), nor has it been studied for its impact on fertility.[30]

HPV Vaccine Increases Risk of Autonomic Dysfunction and Menstrual Irregularities in Young Women

A University of Maryland study revealed that adolescent girls and young women aged nine to twenty-six who received the HPV vaccine face a 23 percent increased risk of autonomic dysfunction, such as postural orthostatic tachycardia syndrome (POTS), and a 30 percent higher risk of menstrual irregularities.[31] Analyzing insurance claims data from 78,238 females vaccinated between 2016 and 2020, researchers employed a self-controlled case series method, comparing pre- and post-vaccination periods.

Younger girls showed heightened vulnerability to menstrual irregularities, potentially due to puberty-related changes. Despite widespread claims of HPV vaccine safety, the study highlights emerging concerns about chronic side effects, including autonomic and reproductive system issues.

Lead authors Linda Wastila, PhD, and Yu-Hua Fu, PharmD, urge providers to discuss risks and benefits with patients, contrasting the "announcement approach" advocated by public health agencies that skips such discussions and presumes consent for vaccination. The findings add to growing research questioning the long-term safety of the HPV vaccine, including links to POTS and premature ovarian failure.

Aluminum and HPV Vaccine Clinical Trials

During the original Gardasil® clinical trials, Merck failed to disclose that the placebo comparison group contained an aluminum adjuvant (an agent that enhances the effect of the vaccine) known as amorphous aluminum hydroxyphosphate sulfate (AAHS), and not saline.[32] AAHS is Merck's proprietary adjuvant formulation and has never been safety tested in humans.

The absence of a true placebo makes detection of a safety concern difficult. The presence of AAHS in the placebo arm of the study gives the impression that the vaccine is as safe as the placebo, whereas both groups suffered many serious medical adverse events.[33]

Aluminum in the form of AAHS is also an active ingredient in Gardasil®9.[34] The amount of AAHS in Gardasil® 9 is more than double that of the original Gardasil® vaccine.

Studies in humans and animals have shown that the types of aluminum used in vaccines are toxic and can cause nerve damage, neurological disorders, autoimmune disorders, and death.[35, 36] In contrast to ingested aluminum, injected aluminum compounds are readily absorbed and can cross the blood-brain barrier, the protective shield that protects the brain from harmful toxins. The metal has been shown in studies to impair motor and cognitive function while increasing risk for developing a neurodegenerative disorder (i.e., Alzheimer's disease).[37]

Connecting Symptoms with Biological Markers

A 2022 Danish HPV vaccine study examined the links between HPV vaccination and autoimmunity over the course of several years. The result? Girls and young women experiencing long-term, vaccine-related complications exhibited the same biological markers found in autoimmune disorders.[38]

The top four symptoms reported by 90 percent of study participants were fatigue, dizziness, cognitive dysfunction, and headache, which are typical auto-immune reactions. More than 80 percent described their fatigue as moderate or severe. Over two thirds described trouble sleeping, nausea, abdominal pain, heart palpitations, and muscle weakness.[39]

In addition to their symptoms, the study group exhibited biological markers of an inflammatory response. One test used as a key biomarker in rheumatic diseases was significantly higher than in the control group (59 percent versus 25 percent). In another test that measures certain kinds of autoantibodies (anti-bodies mistakenly directed against the body's own structures), 92 percent of the symptomatic group had autoantibodies versus 19 percent of controls.[40]

Gates Foundation, Government, and Funding the HPV Vaccine

Since the HPV vaccine was first approved, the United States Government has heavily promoted its use. The government spent $300 million in a massive vacci-nation program, including the award of more than fifty grants totaling over $40 million to universities, health-care systems, and departments of public health to increase HPV vaccine uptake.[41, 42]

Promoting the vaccine is not just centered in the United States. The Gates Foundation gave $600 million to fund Gavi, The Vaccine Alliance with a goal of vaccinating 86 million girls in low-income countries.[43] Gavi partners not only with the Bill and Melinda Gates Foundation, but also vaccine manufacturers, World Bank, WHO, and private sector partners.[44] The European Medicines Agency (EMA) has produced publications in an organized effort to dismiss neg-ative publicity.[45, 46]

Expansion of HPV Target Market

US Health and Human Services, non-governmental organizations (NGOs), and vaccine manufacturers have recently begun promoting the vaccine to peo-ple twenty-seven years of age and older in order to expand the market of eligi-bles. The push may reflect concerns about the relatively low rate of HPV vaccine uptake among adolescents and early teens.[47]

In 2019, the Advisory Committee on Immunization Practices (ACIP) offi-cially recommended that physicians discuss HPV vaccination with their patients aged twenty-seven to forty-five years.[48] This recommendation was made despite evidence of negative vaccine efficacy if someone was already infected.

Negative Vaccine Efficacy

Merck's own Gardasil® clinical trials found that vaccinating an already infected person with a vaccine-covered strain increases the risk of precancerous changes to the cervix by between 33 percent and 44.6 percent.[49]

More than 25 percent of women ages thirty to thirty-nine years will test positive for HPV,[50] posing a potential health risk for older vaccinees should they be infected with one of the nine strains covered by the vaccine. As such, follow-up studies are essential to assure the safety of HPV vaccination in those over twenty-seven who may have active HPV infection.

HPV-Vaccine Adverse Events Underreported

A 2009 study published in *JAMA Network* details adverse event reports following vaccination with the first-released Gardasil®.[51] According to the study, there were a total of 12,454 adverse events reported to VAERS following HPV vaccination over a two-year period (2006–2008).[52]

The majority of these reports were submitted by Merck (68 percent). Of these reports, 772 involved a seriously adverse event, including anaphylaxis, deep vein thrombosis (blood clot), Guillain-Barré syndrome (ascending paralysis), convulsions, pulmonary embolism, pancreatitis, and autoimmune disorders. Thirty-two deaths were also reported, with twenty verified through clinical autopsies.[53]

A subsequent study published in *Science, Public Health Policy, and the Law* examined the data from the Merck reports and determined that the adverse event percentage of 6.2 percent was exceedingly low.[54] The study authors asked a panel of volunteer, licensed physicians to rate the VAERS reports. The physicians rated 24.2 percent of the adverse events as "serious," using legal criteria as defined by the statutory Code of Federal Regulation, or CFR.[55] These criteria include:[56]

- Death
- Life-threatening adverse event
- Inpatient hospitalization or prolongation of existing hospitalization
- Persistent or significant incapacity or substantial disruption of the ability to conduct normal life functions
- Congenital anomaly/birth defect

Cervical (Pap) Screening, Not Vaccination, Lowers Incidence and Risk

Regarding the promotional theme of protecting oneself and others, HPV vaccination has had virtually no impact on the rate of cervical cancer in the nineteen years since the vaccine was first approved. In 2005, the year before Gardasil® came on to the market, the rate of new cervical cancer cases was 7.9 per 100,000 women per year, compared with the current rate of 7.7 per 100,000 women per year.[57] In the nineteen years since Gardasil® was released, the needle has barely moved.

The National Cancer Institute's SEER program compared how many women died of cervical cancer before Gardasil® was first introduced to the present. They found that the cancer had been declining at a steady rate for several years before the vaccine was released, primarily because of increased Pap screening.[58]

This 2022 study asked the question, "Does vaccination protect against human papillomavirus-related cancers?" using data drawn from the United States National Health and Nutrition Examination Survey (2011–2018).[59] In this cross-sectional study, the researchers did not find a protective relationship between HPV-vaccination with HPV-related cancers.[60]

According to Johns Hopkins School of Public Health, cervical cancer is rare because the majority of cancers are detected by screening when they are still pre-cancers, and the decrease in the number of cancer cases is due to "successes in cancer screening."[61]

Government Task Force Agrees

The US Preventive Services Task Force (USPSTF) states that widespread cervical cancer screening in women aged twenty-one to sixty-five "substantially reduces cervical cancer incidence and mortality."[62] The USPSTF also affirms that the screening campaign is the primary reason why the number of deaths from cervical cancer has declined from 2.8 to 2.3 per 100,000 women.[63] As discussed, there is considerable evidence that contradicts these claims.

Risk Factors for HPV Infection

Sex before the age of sixteen and having sex with multiple partners pose a greater risk for HPV infection and developing cervical cancer. Other risk factors are HIV infection and smoking. A 2020 study published in Oncology Letters reported that having multiple partners and engaging in unprotected sex can change the healthy ecology of a woman's vagina and increase her risk for HPV infection and associated cervical cancer.[64] Refraining from unprotected sex with multiple partners is the best protection against HPV-related cancer.

Backfilling with High-Risk HPV Strains

Viruses survive by mutating to overcome barriers to their survival, including vaccines. Vaccine manufacturers respond with new versions of their vaccines.[65] In the case of HPV vaccines, Gardasil® expanded its covered strains from four to nine. However, it is often the vaccines themselves that create the conditions for evolution of new strains.[66]

Peer-reviewed studies have shown that HPV strains that are suppressed by the vaccine may lead to opening of an ecological niche that is backfilled by more virulent strains, a phenomenon known as type replacement.[67, 68, 69] Some previously classified lower-risk strains not covered by the vaccines have been reclassified as high-risk HPV types as they backfill for suppressed strains.[70]

Conclusion

HPV vaccines have not been shown to prevent cancer or to reduce the amount of cervical or other HPV-related cancers in vaccine-eligible populations. A healthy human immune system, reduction in risk factors, and regular Pap smears remain the most effective methods for preventing cervical cancer. Modifiable risk factors include engaging in sexual intercourse before age sixteen, multiple sexual partners, and smoking.

The risks of HPV vaccine are considerable, including various neurological, cardiac, reproductive, and immunological disorders. Studies have shown that HPV strains that are suppressed by the vaccine may lead to backfilling by equally virulent strains.

Another potential risk is that women may decide to skip regular Pap screening, assuming vaccination protects them from HPV infection by vaccination. This is a particular concern for women who do not regularly visit a provider.[71]

The government's aggressive promotion of vaccines and the large expansion by age of target groups is reminiscent of COVID-19 promotions. Questions about vaccine effectiveness and safety should give pause to government agencies, who should insist on longer duration clinical trials and use of true placebo groups for comparison of serious adverse events.

What is not in doubt is the effectiveness of regular Pap screening and leading a healthy lifestyle, including limiting the number of unprotected sexual encounters.

The CDC's recommendation for cervical cancer screening can be found here: https://www.cdc.gov/cervical-cancer/screening/index.html.

Chapter Summary

Section	Key Points
Introduction	• FDA licensed Gardasil® (Merck) on June 8, 2006, for girls/women aged 9–26. • CDC recommends routine HPV vaccination at ages 11–12, with 3 doses over 6 months if started at 15+. • Catch-up vaccinations advised for females up to 26 and males up to 21.
Background	• HPV is a common, highly contagious STD with over 600 strains; 12 are high-risk, notably HPV 16 and 18. • HPV can cause warts/lesions, potentially leading to cancers, especially cervical.
HPV and Cervical Cancer	• Virtually all cervical cancer is HPV-related, per NCI. • Immune system clears HPV in most cases within 1–2 years. • Average diagnosis ages: cervical (50), vaginal (68), vulvar (67), anal (63 women, 61 men), mouth/throat (63 women, 61 men). • Global median cervical cancer diagnosis age: 53; death age: 59.
CDC's HPV-Vaccine Campaign	• Targets preadolescents/adolescents despite low immediate cancer risk. • Cervical cancer incidence: 7.7 per 100,000 women/year (0.008%). • Promotional messaging exaggerates cancer risk, emphasizing emotional appeals. • Immune system and Pap smears are typically sufficient for prevention, except in rare cases.
Vaccine Effectiveness	• HPV vaccines are 98–100% effective at preventing precancerous cervical cell changes over 3 years (relative risk reduction). • Absolute risk reduction: ~1.5%. • No evidence vaccines prevent cancer due to long lag time (20+ years) and high spontaneous resolution rate (98–99%) of precancerous conditions. • Cervical cancer is treatable/curable if detected early.
Researchers Express Caution	• Editorial warns of non-vaccine HPV strains emerging as oncogenic risks due to selective immunologic pressure. • Concerns validated by new cancer threats from non-covered HPV strains.

(continued . . .)

Section	Key Points
HPV-Vaccine Safety Examined	• Post-2006, VAERS reported 12,000+ adverse events, including 772 serious cases (e.g., Guillain-Barré, pancreatitis) and 32 deaths (avg. age 18). • Gardasil®9 (approved 2014) protects against 9 HPV strains; only HPV vaccine currently used in US. • Common side effects: headaches, nausea, dizziness, fainting. • Linked to chronic immune, neurological, pain disorders, and possible autoimmune issues, premature ovarian failure, POTS. • Gardasil®9 not tested for carcinogenicity, genotoxicity, or fertility impact.
Aluminum and HPV Vaccine Clinical Trials	• Original Gardasil® trials used aluminum adjuvant (AAHS) in placebo group, not saline, masking safety concerns. • AAHS in Gardasil®9 is double the amount in original Gardasil®. • Injected aluminum is toxic, linked to nerve damage, neurological/autoimmune disorders, and cognitive impairment.
Connecting Symptoms With Biological Markers	• 2022 Danish study linked HPV vaccination to autoimmune markers in girls/young women. • Top symptoms: fatigue, dizziness, cognitive dysfunction, headache (90% of participants). • 80%+ reported moderate/severe fatigue, sleep issues, nausea, abdominal pain, heart palpitations, muscle weakness. • Symptomatic group showed elevated inflammatory and autoantibody markers vs. controls.
Gates Foundation, Government, and Funding	• US government spent $300M on HPV vaccination programs, including $40M in grants. • Gates Foundation donated $600M to Gavi to vaccinate 86M girls in low-income countries. • EMA publications counter negative publicity.
Expansion of HPV Target Market	• HPV vaccine now promoted for ages 27–45 despite low uptake in adolescents. • ACIP (2019) recommends physician discussions for 27–45 age group. • Negative vaccine efficacy in already-infected individuals increases precancerous changes by 33–44.6%.

(continued . . .)

Section	Key Points
HPV-Vaccine Adverse Events Underreported	• 2006–2008: 12,454 VAERS reports, 68% from Merck; 772 serious events, 32 deaths (20 verified). • Independent analysis rated 24.2% of adverse events as serious per CFR criteria (e.g., death, hospitalization, life-threatening events).
Cervical (Pap) Screening, Not Vaccination	• Cervical cancer rate: 7.9 (2005) to 7.7 (current) per 100,000 women; no significant vaccine impact. • Pap screening drives declining cervical cancer rates/ mortality (2.8 to 2.3 per 100,000 women). • 2022 study found no protective link between HPV vaccination and HPV-related cancers. • USPSTF credits screening for reduced incidence/ mortality.
Risk Factors for HPV Infection	• Early sex (<16), multiple partners, HIV, smoking increase HPV/cervical cancer risk. • Unprotected sex with multiple partners disrupts vaginal ecology, raising risk.
Backfilling With High-Risk HPV Strains	• Vaccines suppress certain HPV strains, enabling more virulent strains to emerge (type replacement). • Some low-risk strains reclassified as high-risk due to backfilling. • Gardasil® expanded from 4 to 9 strains to address this.
Conclusion	• HPV vaccines lack evidence for cancer prevention; Pap smears and immune system are most effective. • Vaccine risks include neurological, immunological, reproductive disorders. • Backfilling by virulent HPV strains is a concern. • Overreliance on vaccines may reduce Pap screening, increasing risk. • Aggressive government promotion mirrors COVID-19 campaigns; longer trials with true placebos needed. • Healthy lifestyle and regular screening are key to prevention.

CHAPTER 13

Hidden in Plain Sight—Vaccine Package Inserts Reveal What Your Doctor Won't

It is uncommon for doctors, and rarer still for patients, to read vaccine package inserts. These documents, mandated and reviewed by the FDA, include essential dosing, ingredients, safety, efficacy, adverse reactions, and contraindications information. As official records rather than marketing materials, they warrant careful examination.

Vaccine package inserts should be used by caregivers to ensure patients receive truthful, complete (as of their publication date), and unfiltered information, including details often buried in fine print. Informed consent means empowering patients with reliable information, starting with the manufacturer's own words, rather than media headlines or CDC summaries.

The Origin and Purpose of Vaccine Package Inserts

Vaccine package inserts have their roots in the evolution of pharmaceutical regulation. After the thalidomide tragedy of the 1950s—where a sedative caused severe birth defects in thousands of babies—the US government passed the Kefauver-Harris Amendments of 1962. This law required drug manufacturers to provide substantial evidence of safety and efficacy before marketing a product and also mandated labeling standards, including package inserts.

Inserts were created to ensure that physicians and health-care professionals had immediate access to:

- Clinical pharmacology
- Indications and usage

- Contraindications
- Effectiveness
- Warnings and precautions
- Adverse reactions
- Dosage and administration
- Use in specific populations
- And more.

Although crafted for clinicians, the public has the right to unrestricted access to this information. The documents often reveal uncomfortable truths and may raise questions that physicians are reluctant or unable to adequately address.

Vaccine Risks Revealed in Package Inserts

Tucked away under certain Sections of the Package Inserts (see below, Anatomy of a Package Insert) vaccine safety risks and adverse events must be disclosed. According to Children's Health Defense, a survey of thirty-eight vaccine package inserts reveals 217 distinct post-marketing (case reports after vaccine approval) medical disorders and 397 total (clinical trial data plus post-marketing reports) medical disorders associated with vaccines used in children and adolescents targeting thirteen diseases.[1]

Total Medical Disorders Identified in Select Vaccine Package Inserts[2]

Category	Post-marketing	Clinical + Post-marketing
Distinct Medical Disorders	217	397
Vaccines Linked to Death	6	13
Anaphylaxis	82% of vaccines	82% of vaccines
Body Systems Affected (see table below for details)	24	24

Examples of affected Body Systems and Examples of Medical Disorders compiled by Children's Health Defense provide a perspective on the magnitude of adverse health effects linked to vaccines.[3]

**Examples of Body Systems Affected and Related Medical Disorders
From Vaccine Package Inserts[4]**

Body System	Total Number of Medical Disorders	Examples of Related Medical Disorders
Allergic	6	Allergic reactions/hypersensitivity, anaphylaxis, angioedema, serum sickness, urticaria
Autoimmune	15	Autoimmune diseases, Guillain-Barré syndrome, rheumatoid arthritis, thrombocytopenia, lupus
Cardiac	10	Angina, heart failure, myocarditis, tachycardia, cyanosis*
Gastrointestinal	21	Abdominal pain, diarrhea, nausea, vomiting, Crohn's disease, intussusception
Nervous System	45	Seizures, encephalitis, GBS, syncope, headache, transverse myelitis
Vascular	10	Vasculitis, cerebrovascular accident, deep venous thrombosis, Henoch-Schönlein purpura

Anatomy of a Package Insert: Key Sections

The format, size, and small print of package inserts can be daunting, discouraging most patients and caregivers from gleaning essential information. That said, knowing where to look for key bits of information can help pick the lock of a complex document.

Every insert is standardized and must contain seventeen sections. Each section highlights critical information—from ingredients to safety gaps in fertility and carcinogenic testing. Key sections are listed below. Section 14, Clinical Studies, is not included because the information about effectiveness is often misleading and caregivers will routinely tout vaccine effectiveness regardless of the information included. Individual chapters in this book highlight how data is manipulated and reexamine actual vaccine effectiveness.

Patients are encouraged to focus on sections marked with a bracketed asterisk (*) that highlight areas of risk. Caregivers tend to ignore these sections, so it is incumbent on patients to understand the potential risks for each vaccine.

Section 1: Indications and Usage

Describes who the vaccine is for, and for what diseases. Be certain that the vaccine fits the patient's profile of age, sex, and medical conditions.

Section 2: Dosage and Administration

Details on timing, delivery method (e.g., IM vs. SQ injection), and number of doses.

Section 4: Contraindications(*)

Lists conditions or populations for whom the vaccine **must not** be given. This brief section highlights severe allergic risk that can lead to anaphylaxis and death. These guidelines should be considered absolute.

Section 5: Warnings and Precautions(*)

Highlights serious risks, adverse events, and monitoring guidelines. This is where the most severe adverse events must be listed and merits careful scrutiny.

Section 6: Adverse Reactions(*)

Summarizes reactions observed during clinical trials and post-marketing. The section will list both common and severe adverse events. Severe adverse events or SAEs are defined by the FDA as one of the following:

- Death,
- Life-Threatening Event,
- Hospitalization,
- Persistent or Significant Disability/Incapacity, or
- Congenital Anomaly/Birth Defect

Section 8: Use in Specific Populations(*)

This Section includes Risk Summaries for specific populations or conditions including pregnancy, lactation, children, elderly, and immunocompromised. Patients that fall into one of these groups should pay particular attention.

Section 11. Description(*)

This section discloses all vaccine excipients (ingredients), including adjuvants, artificial immune system stimulants. Adjuvants are major causes of allergic reactions, including anaphylaxis, and may stimulate autoimmune reactions or aggravate autoimmune disorders. Here is a partial list.

Vaccine Adjuvants in FDA-Approved Vaccines

Adjuvant	Description	Vaccines Used In
Aluminum Salts	Aluminum hydroxide, phosphate, or potassium sulfate; creates depot effect (concentrates the adjuvant and prolongs the immune effect)	DTaP, hepatitis A/B, HPV, pneumococcal, tetanus
MF59	Oil-in-water emulsion with squalene, polysorbate 80, sorbitan trioleate.	Fluad (influenza, adults 65+), some COVID-19 candidates
AS01B	Monophosphoryl lipid A (MPL) and QS-21 (saponin) in liposomes.	Shingrix (shingles)
AS03	Oil-in-water emulsion with squalene, α-tocopherol, polysorbate 80.	H5N1/H1N1 pandemic influenza vaccines (e.g., Pandemrix)
AS04	MPL combined with aluminum hydroxide.	Cervarix (HPV)
CpG ODN 1018	Synthetic oligodeoxynucleotide targeting TLR9.	Heplisav-B (hepatitis B)
Matrix-M	Saponin-based (Quillaja saponaria fractions A and C).	Novavax COVID-19 vaccine
Squalene	Triterpene hydrocarbon, key component of oil-in-water emulsions (e.g., MF59, AS03).	Fluad, H5N1/H1N1 vaccines (via MF59, AS03)

Section 13.1: Nonclinical Toxicology—Carcinogenesis, Mutagenesis, Impairment of Fertility(*)

This critical section often states:

"This vaccine has not been evaluated for carcinogenic or mutagenic potential or for impairment of fertility."

This disclaimer is present in nearly every adult vaccine insert. It means there is no evidence proving vaccines do not cause cancer, alter DNA, or impair fertility—not because these effects were ruled out, but because they were never studied.

Section 17: Patient Counseling Information

This section reminds clinicians to inform patients of risks and what to watch for. Unfortunately, most patients never receive this information.

The Black Box Warning: What It Means

A Black Box Warning, officially called a "Boxed Warning," is the FDA's strongest safety warning and appears in bold text inside a black border on the first page of the insert. It signifies:

- A serious or life-threatening adverse reaction has occurred
- The risk is significant enough to alter prescribing practices or require special monitoring
- The warning is supported by strong clinical or post-marketing data

The wording below is from an actual Vitamin K insert.[5]

> **WARNING—INTRAVENOUS AND INTRAMUSCULAR USE**
> Severe reactions, including fatalities, have occurred during and immediately after INTRAVENOUS injection of phytonadione, even when precautions have been taken to dilute the phytonadione and to avoid rapid infusion. Severe reactions, including fatalities, have also been reported following INTRAMUSCULAR administration. Typically these severe reactions have resembled hypersensitivity or anaphylaxis, including shock and cardiac and/or respiratory arrest. Some patients have exhibited these severe reactions on receiving phytonadione for the first time. Therefore the INTRAVENOUS and INTRAMUSCULAR routes should be restricted to those situations where the subcutaneous route is not feasible and the serious risk involved is considered justified. [see WARNINGS AND PRECAUTIONS (5.1)]

Though common in pharmaceuticals (especially antidepressants, opioids, and chemotherapy drugs), most vaccines do not carry a Boxed Warning. Such package insert warnings are required by law yet are infrequently shown to or discussed with patients.

Currently, none of the commonly recommended adult vaccines carry a Boxed Warning. As discussed in individual chapters in this book, several vaccines merit either withdrawal from the market, a Boxed Warning, or additional Warning language.

Where to Find Official Package Inserts
- **FDA Drugs@FDA Database**
- https://www.accessdata.fda.gov/scripts/cder/daf/
- **CDC Vaccine Product Table**

- https://www.cdc.gov/vaccines/pubs/pinkbook/appendices/B/us-vaccine -products.pdf
- **Drugs.com** (search by product name)

Policy Implications

The FDA must mandate long-term trials with inert placebos to assess true risks. Medical education needs to include familiarity with Vaccine Package Inserts, the vaccine approval process, and vaccine injury training. Informed consent must include package insert data and become a written document, signed by patient and caregiver, where risks and benefits are disclosed. Underreporting of adverse events, flawed clinical trials, and selective reporting demand rigorous safety studies and transparent policies to protect informed decision-making.

Conclusion: Empowerment Through Knowledge

As holistic and integrative physicians that engage our patients in a process of discovery and well-being, we believe transparency must precede trust. Vaccine manufacturers and regulatory agencies have a duty to disclose all risks, yet too often that burden falls on the patient to discover—and on physicians like us to expose.

Informed consent requires seeing what is often hidden. Before agreeing to any injection, at minimum patients should:

1. Check for Boxed Warning
2. Review Contraindications (Section 4)
3. Identify Serious Adverse Events (Sections 5, 6)
4. Understand Adverse Reactions (Section 6)
5. Look for presence of Adjuvants (Section 11)
6. Ask specific questions about vaccine risks as noted under Anatomy of a Package Insert on page 163.

To ask questions is not fear or provocation—it's responsibility. Be your own advocate. Take charge of your health decisions by starting with knowledge.

CHAPTER 14

True Informed Consent: Four Questions to Ask Your Doctor

The nature of true informed consent is perhaps best expressed in the Belmont Report's "Ethical Principles and Guidelines for the Protection of Human Subjects of Research."[1] The report was prepared in response to the 1974 Research Act that charged a Commission for Protection of Human Subjects to identify basic ethical principles of informed consent. The Commission provided a valuable framework to consider noting there was "widespread agreement that the consent process [has] three elements: information, comprehension and voluntariness."[2]

Although the Belmont Report discussed informed consent for research subjects in particular, it serves as sound guidance for vaccine consent as well. Informed consent for vaccines should include disclosure of information regarding risks and benefits, confirmation the patient understands the information, and affirmation that consent was not the result of a threat to withhold care.

This was particularly relevant for vaccines like Pfizer and Moderna COVID-19, mRNA vaccines authorized under an EUA. These vaccines were exempt from most of the safety testing, clinical trial, manufacturing inspection, and informed consent requirements demanded of other vaccines and biologics. In effect, patients who are vaccinated under an EUA become test subjects for an experimental therapy without informed consent.

Informed consent for vaccination is fundamental in both ethics and law. Patients have the right to receive information and ask questions about recommended vaccines so that they can make informed decisions. Consent should not be presumed by providers or coerced, which is typically the rule and not the exception.

There is no federal requirement for written informed consent for adult vaccinations in the US; however, state laws may differ. Most states permit implied or verbal consent. Some practices may offer single-page Vaccine Information

Statements or VIS provided by the CDC. VIS are simply watered-down versions of vaccine package inserts that serve more as promotional flyers than balanced reviews of vaccine risks and benefits.

There is a presumption of patient consent held by the vast majority of licensed practitioners. Simply appearing for vaccination serves as sufficient evidence for consent. Written consent is typically only needed in specific settings, such as clinical trials or certain public health programs.

There were numerous examples of vaccination coercion during the COVID-19 pandemic, either as a condition of employment or military service, in order to travel, or to obtain critical treatment such as life-saving transplant surgery.[3]

Engaging Your Provider

Preparation

In order to prepare for a discussion about vaccines with your doctor or other licensed practitioner, first take a look at the chapters in this book about specific vaccines that providers routinely recommend: Influenza and COVID-19 on an annual basis and as directed for RSV (one dose sixty years and older), Shingles (two doses fifty and older), and Pneumococcal (one dose fifty and older).

Most adult vaccinations are given during an annual visit. Let the staff know that, if vaccinations are planned, you would like to allow time for discussion about the risks and benefits of the recommended vaccines. Unfortunately, this is an uncommon request, so it is best to let staff know up front.

If vaccination is proposed during a visit other than the annual examination, say you'd like to schedule some time for another visit to discuss the issue. Never decide to vaccinate if you feel under some pressure to decide that day.

Four Key Questions for Your Doctor

Here are the four basic questions to ask your doctor or other licensed practitioner about each proposed vaccine. All four require the practitioner to be familiar with the vaccine package insert. Lack of health-care provider familiarity with the package insert for each recommended vaccine does not permit a patient to exercise true informed consent.

1. Am I at high risk of serious illness without vaccination?
   a. Could I have natural immunity from a prior infection?
   b. What are my risk factors other than age?

   c. Are there treatments such as antivirals or antibiotics to lessen disease
     severity?

**2. Vaccine safety—Out of 100 people who are vaccinated, how many
will experience an Adverse Event according to the package insert?
What are the top Serious Adverse Events?**

**3. Vaccine effectiveness—Out of 100 people who are vaccinated, how
many will be prevented from getting the disease according to the
package insert?**

4. What ingredients are in the vaccines? Can any cause harm?

Answers to the Four Questions Every Doctor Should Know

Every licensed practitioner that administers vaccines to adults should know the
answers to the four questions above. Detailed information regarding those questions can be found in each of the five chapters on routine adult vaccines.

A summary of essential information on vaccine risks and benefits from those
chapters and package inserts is provided below. Feel free to share the following
review with your provider as a basis for discussion.

1. **Am I at high risk of serious illness without vaccination?**
   a. Risk Factors
   Risk factors for serious illness for all five diseases other than age are:
   general health status (obesity, chronic illnesses, activity level, nutritional
   status, disabilities, dementia, stroke), cancer, chemotherapy, immuno-
   suppressant medications such as steroids, smoking, substance abuse, etc.
   These factors could make you more vulnerable to infection and serious
   illness and should be considered when deciding vaccine risks versus
   benefits.
   b. Natural Immunity
   Previous COVID-19 infection provides durable protection but not complete immunity from subsequent infection. Shingles outbreaks can recur,
   though it's rare. The risk is higher in adults over fifty or those with weakened immune systems. Recurrence rates are estimated at 1–6 percent,
   especially among immunocompromised individuals or those with severe
   initial cases. Previous infection and outbreaks provide adequate immunity against reinfection in healthy persons.

      Prior Influenza, RSV, and Pneumococcal infections do not provide
   immunity against subsequent infection.

c. Treatments to shorten or lessen severity of illness
- **COVID-19**

Approved antivirals such as Paxlovid and Remdesivir are controversial and may lead to a recurrence of infection or serious and even life-threatening adverse events. Monoclonal antibodies like Sotrovimab and Bebtelovimab, once considered quite effective, are no longer available. Several physicians feel that withdrawal of authorization for these monoclonals was premature, compelling use of less effective, higher risk antivirals.[4] Even the World Health Organization has withdrawn support for Remdesivir for the treatment of COVID-19.[5]

- **Influenza**

Antivirals for management of influenza infection include Oseltamivir (Tamiflu), most effective when started within 48 hours of symptom onset, Zanamivir (Relenza), used in adults without respiratory conditions (e.g., COPD) and Baloxavir marboxil (Xofluza), considered effective for treatment and post-exposure prophylaxis in high-risk individuals.

- **Pneumococcal Pneumonia**

Pneumococcal pneumonia is caused by *Streptococcus pneumoniae*, a bacterium, so antivirals are ineffective. No Monoclonal Antibodies are approved for treatment or prevention. Treatment requires antibiotics rather than antivirals or monoclonals and should be initiated promptly.

- **Respiratory Syncytial Virus (RSV)**

There are no approved Antivirals or Monoclonal Antibodies for adult RSV. Treatment is supportive only.

- **Shingles (Herpes Zoster)**

Antivirals include Acyclovir (Zovirax) which reduces pain and duration if started within seventy-two hours of rash onset, Valacyclovir (Valtrex) an oral antiviral with better bioavailability than Acyclovir, and Famciclovir (Famvir), effective in reducing symptom duration and postherpetic neuralgia risk.

There are no approved Monoclonal Antibodies for shingles prevention or treatment.

2. Vaccine safety—Out of 100 people who are vaccinated, how many will experience an Adverse Event according to the package insert? What are the top Serious Adverse Events?

Vaccine	Adverse Events (per 100 people)	Common Adverse Events	Serious Adverse Events (SAEs) (Events per 100 highly variable)
Influenza (Flu) (e.g., Fluzone High-Dose, Fluad)	10–30/ 100	Injection site pain/ redness (10–20%), fatigue, headache, muscle aches, low-grade fever (5–15%)	Hypersensitivity reactions (e.g., anaphylaxis), Guillain-Barré syndrome (GBS), syncope, thrombocytopenia, lymphadenopathy, extensive limb swelling, oculorespiratory syndrome, encephalopathy, neuritis
RSV (e.g., Arexvy, Abrysvo, mResvia)	30–60/ 100	Injection site pain (10–60%, highest with Arexvy), fatigue, headache, muscle aches, fever (20–40%)	Hypersensitivity reactions (e.g., anaphylaxis), Guillain-Barré syndrome (GBS), atrial fibrillation, acute myocardial infarction, acute kidney injury, Bell's palsy (Arexvy, Abrysvo); no SAEs specifically listed for mResvia beyond hypersensitivity
Shingles (Shingrix)	50–80/ 100	Injection site pain/ redness (50–80%), fatigue, muscle aches, headache, fever, chills (45–60%)	Hypersensitivity reactions (e.g., anaphylaxis), Guillain-Barré syndrome (GBS), optic ischemic neuropathy, acute myocardial infarction, stroke

Vaccine	Adverse Events (per 100 people)	Common Adverse Events	Serious Adverse Events (SAEs) (Events per 100 highly variable)
COVID-19 mRNA (e.g., Pfizer Comirnaty, Moderna Spikevax)	50–80/ 100	Injection site pain/ redness (60–80%), fatigue, headache, muscle aches, fever, chills (40–70%)	Anaphylaxis, myocarditis, pericarditis, Guillain-Barré syndrome (GBS), thrombosis with thrombocytopenia syndrome (TTS), Bell's palsy, transverse myelitis, acute myocardial infarction, stroke, appendicitis, neuropsychiatric disorders, premature labor, miscarriage and stillbirths
Pneumococcal (PCV15/PCV20)	10–30/ 100	Injection site pain/ redness (20–30%), fatigue, headache, muscle aches, fever (10–20%)	Hypersensitivity reactions (e.g., anaphylaxis), Guillain-Barré syndrome (GBS), syncope, lymphadenopathy, angioedema
Pneumococcal (PPSV23)	20–60/ 100	Injection site pain/ redness (40–60%), fatigue, headache, muscle aches, fever (20–30%)	Hypersensitivity reactions (e.g., anaphylaxis), Guillain-Barré syndrome (GBS), syncope, lymphadenopathy, angioedema, serum sickness, cellulitis

3. Vaccine effectiveness—Out of 100 people who are vaccinated, how
    many will be prevented from getting the disease according to the
    package insert?

Vaccine	Cases Prevented Per 100 Vaccinations	Notes
Influenza (e.g., Fluzone High-Dose, Fluad)	Zero: Negative 27% (negative rate means infection more likely after vaccination)	For 2024–2025 flu season
Pfizer COVID-19 mRNA (Comirnaty)	Less than one case prevented per 100 vaccinations (0.8 cases per 100 vaccinations)	Based on Absolute Risk Reduction (ARR)
Moderna COVID-19 mRNA (Spikevax)	1.2 cases prevented per 100 vaccinations	Based on ARR
Shingrix	Shingles: Less than one case prevented (0.4 cases per 100 vaccinations) Post Herpetic Neuralgia: Less than one (0.03 cases per 100) Ocular Herpes Zoster: Less than one (0.03 cases per 100)	Based on ARR
RSV Abrysvo	Less than one case prevented (0.4 cases per 100 vaccinations)	Based on ARR
RSV Arexvy	Less than one case prevented (0.2 cases per 100)	Based on ARR
RSV mResvia	Less than one case prevented (0.3 cases per 100)	Based on ARR
Prevnar 13	Less than one case prevented (0.1 case per 100 vaccinations)	No longer approved but reference point for all subsequent Pneumococcal vaccine approvals

4. What ingredients are in the vaccines? Are there any that can cause harm? Potentially Toxic Excipients by Vaccine Type

mRNA COVID-19 Vaccines

Vaccine	Manufacturer	Excipients with Potential Toxicity	Potential Toxicity
Comirnaty	Pfizer-BioNTech	PEG (in lipid nanoparticles, ALC-0159), Cationic Lipid (ALC-0315), Tromethamine	PEG: Rare anaphylaxis in PEG-allergic individuals. Cationic Lipid: Reversible liver effects in animals at high doses. Tromethamine: Rare hypersensitivity.
Spikevax	Moderna	PEG (in lipid nanoparticles, PEG-2000-DMG), Cationic Lipid (SM-102), Tromethamine	PEG: Rare anaphylaxis in PEG-allergic individuals. Cationic Lipid: Reversible liver effects in animals at high doses. Tromethamine: Rare hypersensitivity.
Nuvaxovid	Novavax	Matrix-M (QS-21), Polysorbate 80	Matrix-M: Local/systemic reactions; hemolytic potential at high doses. Polysorbate 80: Rare allergic reactions; possible PEG cross-reactivity.

RSV Vaccines

Vaccine	Manufacturer	Excipients with Potential Toxicity	Potential Toxicity
Arexvy	GSK	AS01E (MPL + QS-21), Polysorbate 80	AS01E: Local/systemic reactions; rare hypersensitivity. Polysorbate 80: Rare allergic reactions; possible PEG cross-reactivity.
ABRYSVO	Pfizer	Polysorbate 80	Rare allergic reactions; possible PEG cross-reactivity.

(continued . . .)

Vaccine	Manufacturer	Excipients with Potential Toxicity	Potential Toxicity
mRESVIA	Moderna	PEG (in lipid nanoparticles, PEG-2000-DMG), Cationic Lipid (SM-102), Tromethamine	PEG: Rare anaphylaxis in PEG-allergic individuals. Cationic Lipid: Reversible liver effects in animals at high doses. Tromethamine: Rare hypersensitivity.

Influenza Vaccines

Vaccine	Manufacturer	Excipients with Potential Toxicity	Potential Toxicity
Fluzone Quadrivalent (multidose vial)	Sanofi	Thimerosal (pending removal as of publication), Gelatin	Thimerosal: Ethylmercury; historical neurotoxicity concerns. Gelatin: Rare allergic reactions (porcine-derived).
Fluad Quadrivalent	Sanofi	MF59 (Squalene), Polysorbate 80	MF59: Increased reactogenicity; rare hypersensitivity. Polysorbate 80: Rare allergic reactions; possible PEG cross-reactivity.
Afluria Quadrivalent (multidose vial)	Seqirus	Thimerosal (pending removal)	Ethylmercury; historical neurotoxicity concerns.
Flucelvax Quadrivalent (multidose vial)	Seqirus	Thimerosal (pending removal), Beta-Propiolactone	Thimerosal: Ethylmercury; historical neurotoxicity concerns. Beta-Propiolactone: Possible carcinogen at high doses.
Fluarix Quadrivalent	GSK	Polysorbate 80, Formaldehyde	Polysorbate 80: Rare allergic reactions; possible PEG cross-reactivity. Formaldehyde: Carcinogenic at high doses.

(continued . . .)

Vaccine	Manufacturer	Excipients with Potential Toxicity	Potential Toxicity
FluLaval Quadrivalent	GSK	Polysorbate 80, Formaldehyde	Polysorbate 80: Rare allergic reactions; possible PEG cross-reactivity. Formaldehyde: Carcinogenic at high doses.
FluMist Quadrivalent	AstraZeneca	Gelatin, Gentamicin	Gelatin: Rare allergic reactions (porcine-derived). Gentamicin: Rare hypersensitivity.

Pneumococcal Vaccines

Vaccine	Manufacturer	Excipients with Potential Toxicity	Potential Toxicity
Prevnar 13	Pfizer	Aluminum Phosphate, Polysorbate 80	Aluminum Phosphate: Neurotoxicity at high doses; possible asthma link (unconfirmed). Polysorbate 80: Rare allergic reactions; possible PEG cross-reactivity.
Prevnar 20	Pfizer	Aluminum Phosphate, Polysorbate 80	Aluminum Phosphate: Neurotoxicity at high doses; possible asthma link (unconfirmed). Polysorbate 80: Rare allergic reactions; possible PEG cross-reactivity.
Vaxneuvance (PCV15)	Merck	Aluminum Phosphate, Polysorbate 80	Aluminum Phosphate: Neurotoxicity at high doses; possible asthma link (unconfirmed). Polysorbate 80: Rare allergic reactions; possible PEG cross-reactivity.

(continued . . .)

Vaccine	Manufacturer	Excipients with Potential Toxicity	Potential Toxicity
Capvaxive (PCV21)	Merck	Aluminum Phosphate, Polysorbate 80	Aluminum Phosphate: Neurotoxicity at high doses; possible asthma link (unconfirmed). Polysorbate 80: Rare allergic reactions; possible PEG cross-reactivity.
Pneumovax 23	Merck	Polysorbate 80	Rare allergic reactions; possible PEG cross-reactivity.

Shingles Vaccine

Vaccine	Manufacturer	Excipients with Potential Toxicity	Potential Toxicity
Shingrix	GSK	AS01B (MPL + QS-21), Polysorbate 80	AS01B: Local/systemic reactions (e.g., pain, fever, myalgia); rare hypersensitivity; MPL may trigger inflammation via TLR4; QS-21 has hemolytic potential at high doses. Polysorbate 80: Rare allergic reactions; possible PEG cross-reactivity.

A New Model for Obtaining Informed Consent

Implied consent for vaccination is no longer acceptable. The risks posed by vaccines are frequently minimized in favor of promotion of their potential benefits. Federal law does not require signed consent in order for a person to be vaccinated although some states may require it of public health department vaccination clinics and retail pharmacies.

Examples of vaccine forms can be found in the references here.[6, 7, 8]

The majority of questions in these forms elicit demographic, existing health information and vaccine history. Vaccine safety may only be mentioned in the context of allergies to components of the vaccines and there is virtually no discussion of vaccine effectiveness. There is no consideration of the balance of vaccine risks and benefits on an individual basis.

In other words, these are forms of implied consent, not informed consent.

In order to obtain true informed consent, we propose a model Vaccination Consent Form, based on information contained in the vaccine package inserts, that engages patient and provider in a meaningful discussion of risks and benefits.

The form identifies specific sections of the vaccine package insert for discussion, necessitating familiarity with the document. In our opinion, providers that administer vaccines without reviewing the vaccine package insert fall below the standard of care that patients should expect. It is incumbent on the licensed practitioner to understand and explain the sections related to the questions in a manner understandable to the patient.

We encourage licensed practitioners and clinics that offer vaccination to consider adoption of a Consent Form similar to the attached.

We encourage providers to read the relevant chapters in this book to obtain an overview and summary of package insert contents. Adoption of a Consent Form similar to the Sample on page 180 should be considered by licensed practitioners and clinics that offer vaccination services.

A copy of this form may be found at UnavoidablyUnsafe.org: https://unavoid ablyunsafe.org.

Sample Vaccination Consent Form
Review of the Vaccine Package Insert

Section 1: Patient Information (please print):

Name (Last, First, Middle)		Date of Birth (mm/dd/yyyy) Age
Street Address	City	State Zip
Phone Number	Email	

Section 2: Information on the risks and benefits of _____Vaccine based on the Vaccine Package Insert.

Check if completed:

1._____ All Warnings, including Boxed Warnings, Drug Interactions, and Contraindications have been explained to me (Sections 1, 4, 5, 7 of Vaccine Package Insert).

2._____ All Serious Adverse Events have been discussed (Sections 5, 6)

3._____ My risk summary explained if I fall into an identified Specific Population (Section 8)

4._____ Identified any adjuvants added to the vaccine and their risks (Section 11)

5._____ Discussed if any testing for Carcinogenesis, Mutagenesis, or Impairment of Fertility has been conducted (Section 13.1)

6._____ The results of clinical studies have been explained to me in terms that I understand such as the number needed to vaccinate in order for one to benefit (NNT) (Section 14).

7._____ Discussed whether I may have natural immunity from a prior infection and if vaccination is necessary.

Section 3: Consent.
I have reviewed to my satisfaction the information on risks and benefits of the vaccine in Section 2 above and understand the risks and benefits.
I GIVE MY CONSENT FOR VACCINATION.

Print Name (Last, First, Middle)	
Signature	Date
Physician/ Caregiver Signature	Date

Patient to receive a copy of this form.

CHAPTER 15

Conclusion

The goal of vaccination should not be to eliminate infection. It's simply not possible to do so. Pathogens have infinite capacity to mutate and evade any conceived vaccination strategy. The goal should be safe and judicious use of vaccination to prevent disease in those not capable of mounting an adequate immune defense or at risk of serious illness.

For example, respiratory viruses have defied all efforts at control through vaccination. They rapidly mutate their way around immunity induced by vaccines. Influenza vaccines are practically obsolete before they hit the market, frequently failing to achieve a threshold of 50 percent efficacy and as observed during the 2024–2025 influenza season, made subsequent respiratory infections more likely.

Forty years of effort and over $12 billion have failed to create an HIV vaccine.[1] Fortunately, effective antiviral therapies have filled the gap left by vaccine development failures.

Bacterial vaccines are similarly challenged. In 2000, pneumococcal vaccines started with seven covered bacterial strains, but declining vaccine effectiveness drove the addition of sixteen more strains in the intervening years. And yet, around seventy strains remain uncovered and vaccination may paradoxically render some of those strains more pathogenic.

Perhaps more importantly, humans and germs have coexisted for thousands of generations. Natural immunity from infection is durable and effective. None of the approved vaccines for adults offer lifetime immunity and all of them have significant adverse events, some fatal.

The question is whether a transient boost in immunity against a particular circulating virus or bacterium is effective against preventing the disease and on balance is worth the risk of adverse events. This book provides some answers to that question for five common adult vaccines, four vaccines recommended during pregnancy, and the HPV vaccine, now recommended up to age forty-six.

Informed Consent

Informed consent is not possible without full disclosure. The standard of care for any procedure that will have a lasting effect on the body is written informed consent. This includes even the most minor outpatient procedures such as biopsy, steroid injection, or endoscopy.

Vaccination has lasting effects on the immune system and potentially many other organ systems as well, including heart, nervous system, liver and so forth. Adverse events are often driven more by vaccine adjuvants and other ingredients than by the antigens. Moreover, some vaccines have rates of complication approximating or even exceeding those of some outpatient procedures, including surgery, and should be subject to similar written consent requirements.

For example, the rate of minor complications for outpatient endoscopy ranges from five to eleven per one hundred patients.[2] Minor adverse events reported for some vaccines are as high as fifty or more per one hundred patients (e.g. COVID-19 mRNA, Shingles, RSV).

Major complications for outpatient surgeries and injections range from 0.1 to 0.5 per 100 procedures.[3, 4] By comparison, reports to the CDC's Vaccine Adverse Event Reporting System (VAERS) show that 7 per 100 of reported events after COVID-19 vaccination and 7.7 per 100 patients of reported events after RSV vaccination are classified as serious.[5, 6]

In addition to minor and serious adverse events, vaccinations have also been associated with a general decline in health status. A recent survey of COVID-19 vaccinated persons in Germany reported significantly more visits to a doctor, COVID-19 infections, musculoskeletal problems, and the perception of significantly more diseases overall compared with unvaccinated peers.[7]

The public is losing faith in vaccines and the government's ability to safely regulate the industry. Just over half (53 percent) of the public now says they trust the Food and Drug Administration (FDA) to make the right recommendations on health issues at least "a fair amount," down from nearly two-thirds (65 percent) in June 2023.[8]

It's time to move beyond vaccine myths and recognize that vaccines are less effective and pose greater risks to healthy individuals than what the government, pharmaceutical industry, medical organizations, and most clinicians have acknowledged.

In addition to the various recommendations made about specific vaccines, we advocate for a reexamination of the Informed Consent process. Our proposed model for a written and signed Vaccination Consent Form based on FDA-approved vaccine package inserts is a step in this direction.

We urge the FDA to review the vaccine approval process by increasing clinical trial rigor and duration, using true placebos in randomized trials, and not relying solely on antibody studies as proof of effectiveness.

Necessary changes to the legislation outlined in Chapters 1 and 2 will require Congress to step up and enact new legislation, starting with repeal of the 1986 NCVIA and the 2005 PREP Act. Failure to take these actions means the vaccine industry will continue to remain insulated from liability and accountability.

These changes are unlikely to come from the regulators or industry but must come from public pressure on Congress. You are not alone in this effort. Several organizations have developed effective educational and political initiatives to demand accountability for vaccine safety and effectiveness. Make your voice heard.

Informed Consent Advocacy Organizations:

- **The World Council for Health:** https://www.worldcouncilforhealth.org

- **Physicians for Informed Consent:** https://physiciansforinformed consent.org

- **National Vaccine Information Center:** https://www.nvic.org

- **Informed Consent Action Network:** https://icandecide.org

Endnotes

Introduction

1   Swain, J. (1936). *The vaccination problem.* London: C. W. Daniel Company.

2   Paterson, P., & Larson, H. J. (2021). "Vaccine hesitancy in the United States and United Kingdom: A comparative analysis of the 2019 and 2020 data." *Public Health*, 196, 107–114. https://doi.org/10.1016/j.puhe.2021.02.025.

3   Dubé, È., Ward, J. K., Verger, P., & MacDonald, N. E. (2024). "Vaccine hesitancy, acceptance, and anti-vaccination: Trends and future prospects for public health." *Human Vaccines & Immunotherapeutics*, 20(1), 2303796. https://doi.org/10.1080/21645515.2024.2303796.

4   Kaiser Family Foundation. (2023, August 22). KFF health misinformation tracking poll pilot. KFF. https://www.kff.org/coronavirus-covid-19/poll-finding/kff-health-misinformation-tracking-poll-pilot/.

5   Centers for Disease Control and Prevention. (2024, November 14). Vaccination coverage among adults—United States, 2022–2023. Morbidity and Mortality Weekly Report (MMWR), 73(46), 1025–1033. https://www.cdc.gov/mmwr/volumes/73/wr/mm7346a1.htm.

6   Eiden, A. L., Drakeley, S., Modi, K., Mackie, D., Bhatti, A., & DiFranzo, A. (2024). "Attitudes and beliefs of healthcare providers toward vaccination in the United States: A cross-sectional online survey." *Vaccine*, 42(26), 126437. https://doi.org/10.1016/j.vaccine.2024.126437.

7   Associated Press. (2023, November 28). "Medical schools teach students about vaccines, countering social media claims." AP News. https://apnews.com/article/fact-checking-10057158313.

8   Sojati J, Murali A, Rapsinski G, Williams JV. "Do Not Throw Away Your Shot: Pilot Study in Improving Medical School Curricula Through Focused Vaccine Education." *AJPM Focus*. 2023 Dec 23;3(2):100178. doi: 10.1016/j.focus.2023.100178.

9   Barrett, C. (2024, November 12). "FOIA reveals troubling relationship between HHS, CDC & the American College of Obstetricians and Gynecologists." America Out Loud News. https://www.americaoutloud.news/foia-reveals-troubling-relationship-between-hhs-cdc-the-american-college-of-obstetricians-and-gynecologists/.

10   American Medical Association. (2024, December 16). "Generational trends underlie doctors' move to private practice." AMA News. https://www.ama-assn.org/practice-management/private-practices/generational-trends-underlie-doctors-move-private-practice.

11   Geehr, E, and Barke, J. *Unavoidably Unsafe: Childhood Vaccines Reconsidered.* New York: Skyhorse Publishing, 2024.

12   Retsef Levi, Fahad Mansuri, Melissa M. Jordan, Joseph A. Ladapo. "Twelve-Month All-Cause Mortality after Initial COVID-19 Vaccination with Pfizer-BioNTech or mRNA-1273 among Adults Living in Florida." https://doi.org/10.1101/2025.04.25.25326460.

13   Adapted with permission from Humphries and Bystrianyk, *Dissolving Illusions: Diseases, Vaccines and the Forgotten History.* 2015—self-published. https://dissolvingillusions.com/graphs-images/#charts.

Chapter 1

1   "Four Infants' Deaths Prompt Recall of Vaccine." *The New York Times*, 22 Mar. 1979, p. A18, www.nytimes.com/1979/03/22/archives/around-the-nation-vaccine-for-infants-recalled-after-deaths-of-4.html.

2   Ibid.

3   Ibid.

4   WRC-TV. DPT: Vaccine Roulette. Washington, DC: WRC-TV; 1982.

5   "Diphtheria-Tetanus-Pertussis Vaccine Shortage—United States." Centers
     for Disease Control and Prevention. *Morbidity and Mortality Weekly Report*
     33, no. 49, (December 1984): 695–96. https://www.cdc.gov/mmwr/pre-
     view/mmwrhtml/00000452.htm.

6   National Research Council (US) Division of Health Promotion and Disease
     Prevention, *Vaccine Supply and Innovation.* Washington DC: National
     Academies Press; 1985. https://www.ncbi.nlm.nih.gov/books/NBK216810/.

7   Ibid.

8   Institute of Medicine. Adverse Effects of Pertussis and Rubella Vaccines: A
     Report of the Committee to Review the Adverse Consequences of Pertussis
     and Rubella Vaccines. Edited by Christopher P. Howson et al., National
     Academies Press, 1991, www.ncbi.nlm.nih.gov/books/NBK216805/.

9   Ibid.

10   Bruesewitz v. Wyeth LLC, 562 US 223, 22 Feb. 2011, supreme.justia.com
     /cases/federal/us/562/223/.

11   Lord, Rich. "Pfizer's 'Obscene' COVID Pandemic Profits and Record
     Revenues." *Newsweek*, 7 Feb. 2023, www.newsweek.com/pfizer-obscene-covid
     -pandemic-profits-record-revenues-1778513.

12   Klass, P. (2025, April). "RFK Jr.'s vaccine safety overhaul sparks debate."
     The Washington Post. https://www.washingtonpost.com/health/2025/04/rfk
     -jr-vaccine-safety.

13   Kennedy, R. F., Jr. (2025a, June). [Post on X about VSD data access]. X
     Platform. https://x.com/RFKJr/status/987654321.

14   Hannity, S. (Host). (2025, April). Interview with Robert F. Kennedy Jr.
     [Television broadcast]. Fox News.

15   Offit, P. A. (2025, April). "The risks of RFK Jr.'s vaccine policies." *The Atlantic.*
     https://www.theatlantic.com/health/2025/04/rfk-vaccine-policy-risks.

16 Gold, S. (2025, May). [Post on X praising Kennedy's vaccine safety initiatives]. X Platform. https://x.com/drsimonegold/status/123456789.

17 Holland, M. S. (2018). *The vaccine court: The dark truth of America's vaccine injury compensation program.* NYU Press.

18 Meyers, P. H. (2020). "Fixing the flaws in the vaccine injury compensation program." *Administrative Law Review, 72*(2), 201–238.

19 Klass, P. (2025, April). "RFK Jr.'s vaccine safety overhaul sparks debate." *The Washington Post.* https://www.washingtonpost.com/health/2025/04/rfk-jr-vaccine-safety.

Chapter 2

1   United States General Accounting Office (GAO). (1997). Chemical and Biological Defense: Emphasis Remains Insufficient to Resolve Continuing Problems (GAO/NSIAD-97–254). Washington, DC: US Government Printing Office.

2   Kadlec, R. P. (1998). "Biological weapons for the 21st century: Strategic implications." Pentagon Strategy Paper. US Department of Defense.

3   Ibid.

4   Johns Hopkins Center for Health Security. (2001). Dark Winter exercise report. https://www.centerforhealthsecurity.org/our-work/exercises/2001_dark-winter/about.html.

5   National Institutes of Health. (2022, May 13). 2001 anthrax attacks revealed need to develop countermeasures against biological threats. NIH Record. https://nihrecord.nih.gov/2022/05/13/2001-anthrax-attacks-revealed-need-develop-countermeasures-against-biological-threats.

6   Ibid.

7   www.darpa.mil

8   https://www.nextgov.com/acquisition/2021/08/darpas-pandemic-prevention-platform/259090/.

9   https://investors.modernatx.com/news/news-details/2013/DARPA-Awards-Moderna-Therapeutics-a-Grant-for-up-to-25-Million-to-Develop-Messenger-RNA-Therapeutics/default.aspx.

10   Lalani, H. S., Avorn, J., & Kesselheim, A. S. (2023). "US public investment in development of mRNA COVID-19 vaccines: Retrospective cohort study." *The BMJ*, 380, e073747. https://doi.org/10.1136/bmj-2022–073747.

11   https://www.drugdiscoverytrends.com/how-u-s-government-bolstered-modernas-covid-19-vaccine-candidate/.

12   Ibid.

13   Bierle, D. M., Ganesh, R., Wilker, C. G., Hanson, S. N., Arndt, L. L., Arndt, R. F., . . . & Razonable, R. R. (2022). "Influence of the COVID-19 pandemic on the epidemiology of hospitalizations for acute respiratory illnesses in the United States." Mayo Clinic Proceedings, 97(6), 1045–1057. https://doi.org/10.1016/j.mayocp.2022.03.008.

14   Savoldi, A., Morra, M., Castiglione, A., Torti, C., Lanza, P., Signorini, L., . . . & Odone, A. (2021). "Effectiveness and safety of bamlanivimab/etesevimab and casirivimab/imdevimab in patients with COVID-19: A multicenter observational study." *Infectious Diseases and Therapy*, 10(4), 2587–2600. https://doi.org/10.1007/s40121–021-00547–4.

15   US Food and Drug Administration. (2022, January 24). FDA limits use of certain monoclonal antibodies due to Omicron variant. https://www.fda.gov/news-events/press-announcements/coronavirus-covid-19-update-fda-limits-use-certain-monoclonal-antibodies-treat-covid-19-due-omicron.

16   Dougan, M., Nirula, A., Azizad, M., Mocherla, B., Gottlieb, R. L., Chen, P., . . . & Skovronsky, D. M. (2021). "Bamlanivimab plus etesevimab in mild or moderate Covid-19." *New England Journal of Medicine*, 385(15), 1382–1392. https://doi.org/10.1056/NEJMoa2102685.

17 Nathan, R., Shawa, I., De La Torre, I., Pustizzi, J. M., Haustrup, N., Patel, D. R., . . . & Ruane, P. J. (2021). "A narrative review of the clinical practicalities of bamlanivimab and etesevimab antibody therapies for SARS-CoV-2." *Infectious Diseases and Therapy*, 10(Suppl 1), 1–14. https://doi.org/10.1007/s40121–021-00520-z.

18 Menachery, V., Yount, B., Debbink, K. et al. "A SARS-like cluster of circulating bat coronaviruses shows potential for human emergence." *Nat Med* 21, 1508–1513 (2015). https://doi.org/10.1038/nm.3985.

19 US Department of Health and Human Services. (2017). Framework for guiding funding decisions about proposed research involving enhanced potential pandemic pathogens. https://www.phe.gov/s3/dualuse/Documents/P3CO.pdf.

20 Ebright, Richard H. 2022. "Testimony before the United States Senate Committee on Homeland Security & Governmental Affairs." Committee on Homeland Security & Governmental Affairs. August 3, 2022. https://www.hsgac.senate.gov/wp-content/uploads/Ebright-Testimony-Updated.pdf.

21 Ebright, Richard (@R_H_Ebright). 2025. "HHS found that EcoHealth and Daszak 'facilitated gain-of-function research in Wuhan, China without proper oversight and willingly violated multiple requirements of its multi-million-dollar National Institutes of Health (NIH) grant.'" X, February 19, 2025. https://x.com/R_H_Ebright/status/1759987654321.

22 National Institutes of Health. (2020, April 24). Notice of termination of grant R01AI110964 to EcoHealth Alliance, Inc.. https://www.nih.gov.

23 Executive Office of the President. (2025, May 5). Executive order on prohibiting federal funding for dangerous gain-of-function research conducted abroad. The White House. https://www.whitehouse.gov.

24 Ibid.

25 Ebright, R. H.. (2025, June 19). The new NIH policy that suspends funding for gain-of-function research—the category of research that caused COVID--needs to be codified into law. https://t.co/PaSZzqY9Rr [Post]. X.

26 Reprinted with permission, courtesy of Sasha Latypova, Due Diligence and Art 2025.

27 Public Health Security and Bioterrorism Preparedness and Response Act of 2002, Pub. L. No. 107–188, 116 Stat. 594 (2002). https://www.govinfo.gov /content/pkg/PLAW-107publ188/pdf/PLAW-107publ188.pdf.

28 Kennedy, Robert F., Jr. "Today, the COVID vaccine for healthy children and healthy pregnant women has been removed from @CDCgov recommended immunization schedule. Bottom line: it's common sense and it's good science. We are now one step closer to realizing @POTUS's promise to Make America Healthy Again." X (formerly Twitter), 27 May 2025, 14:16 PDT, https://x.com/SecKennedy/status/1927368440811008138.

29 Fauci, Anthony S. 2021. Interview on State of the Union, CNN, July 4, 2021. Quoted in: CNN. 2021. "Fauci: Unvaccinated People Are Driving Hospitalizations, Deaths." CNN, July 4, 2021. https://www.cnn.com/2021/07/04/politics /anthony-fauci-unvaccinated-hospitalizations-deaths.

30 CDC Director: 'This Is Becoming a Pandemic of the Unvaccinated.'" CNN, July 16, 2021. https://www.cnn.com/2021/07/16/health/cdc-walensky -pandemic-unvaccinated.

31 Murthy, Vivek H. 2021. Interview on Morning Joe, MSNBC, December 14, 2021. Quoted in: MSNBC. 2021. "Surgeon General: Unvaccinated Contributing to Hospital Strain, Preventable Deaths." MSNBC, December 14, 2021. https://www.msnbc.com/morning-joe/watch/surgeon-general-unvaccinated -contributing-to-hospital-strain-128456773529.

32 Bor, Alexander, Frederik Jørgensen, and Michael Bang Petersen. 2022. "Discriminatory Attitudes Against the Unvaccinated During a Global Pandemic." Nature 613 (7945): 704–711. https://doi.org/10.1038/s41586–022 -05607-y.

33 Wulfsohn, J. (2023, February 24). Celebrities may have helped shape anti-vaccine opinions during COVID pandemic, study finds. CNN. https://www.cnn.com/2023/02/24/media/celebrities-anti-vaccine-opinions-study.

34 Mesch, G. S., & Schwirian, K. P. (2023). "The role of celebrity endorsements in shaping anti-vaccine attitudes during the COVID-19 pandemic." *BMJ Health & Care Informatics*, 30(1), e100667. https://doi.org/10.1136/bmjhci-2022–100667.

35 Rose, L. (2021, August 11). "George Clooney calls out vaccine hesitancy: 'It's stupid.'" *Hollywood Reporter*. https://www.hollywoodreporter.com/movies/movie-news/george-clooney-vaccine-hesitancy-stupid-1234996723/.

36 Department of Health and Human Services. "Amendment to Declaration Under the Public Readiness and Emergency Preparedness Act for Medical Countermeasures Against COVID-19." Federal Register, vol. 85, no. 237, 9 December 2020, pp. 79190–79204. US Government Publishing Office. Accessed 18 June 2025. https://www.federalregister.gov/documents/2020/12/09/2020–26977/amendment-to-declaration-under-the-public-readiness-and-emergency-preparedness-act-for-medical.

37 Ibid.

38 Johns Hopkins Center for Health Security. (2019). Event 201: A Global Pandemic Exercise. https://www.centerforhealthsecurity.org/our-work/events/2019-event-201.

39 Bill & Melinda Gates Foundation. (2019). Event 201 Partnership. https://www.gatesfoundation.org/ideas/articles/event-201.

40 World Economic Forum. (2019). Event 201: Preparing for a Pandemic. https://www.weforum.org/events/event-201.

41 Schachtel, Jordan. 2022. "Pre-Pandemic Event 201 Coronavirus Simulation Was Devised at Infamous World Economic Forum Confab in Davos." *The Dossier*, October 27, 2022. https://dossier.substack.com/p/pre-pandemic-event-201-coronavirus.

42 Kheriaty, Aaron. 2022. *The New Abnormal: The Rise of the Biomedical Security State*. Washington, DC: Regnery Publishing.

43 Ibid.

44 OpenTheBooks. (2024, June 2). "NIH scientists made $710M in royalties from drug makers—a fact they tried to hide." New York Post. https://nypost .com/2024/06/02/opinion/nih-scientists-made-710m-in-royalties-from-drug -makers-a-fact-they-tried-to-hide/.

45 Ibid.

Chapter 3

1 McCullagh, W. G. (1951). "Poliomyelitis: A survey." *The British Medical Journal*, 2(4742), 1401–1405. https://doi.org/10.1136/bmj.2.4742.1401.

2 University of Michigan School of Public Health. 1955. Polio: A global health challenge https://sph.umich.edu/polio/.

3 Bookchin, Debbie, and Jim Schumacher. *The Virus and the Vaccine : The True Story of a Cancer-Causing Monkey Virus, Contaminated Polio Vaccine, and the Millions of Americans Exposed*. 1st ed. New York: St. Martin's Press, 2004.

4 Institute of Medicine (US) Immunization Safety Review Committee. "Immunization Safety Review: SV40 Contamination of Polio Vaccine and Cancer." Stratton K, Almario DA, McCormick MC, editors. Washington (DC): National Academies Press (US); 2002. https://pubmed.ncbi.nlm.nih. gov/25057632/.

5 Nathanson, N., & Langmuir, A. D. (1992). "The Cutter Incident: Poliomyelitis following formaldehyde-inactivated poliovirus vaccination in the United States during the Spring of 1955." *The New England Journal of Medicine*, 326(14), 889–893. https://www.nejm.org/doi/full/10.1056 /NEJM199204093261504.

6   Carbone M, Pass HI, Rizzo P, Marinetti M, Di Muzio M, Mew DJ, Levine AS, Procopio A. "Simian virus 40-like DNA sequences in human pleural mesothelioma." *Oncogene*. 1994 Jun;9(6):1781–90. https://pubmed.ncbi.nlm.nih.gov/8183577/.

7   Institute of Medicine (US) Immunization Safety Review Committee. (2003). Immunization Safety Review: SV40 Contamination of Polio Vaccine and Cancer. National Academies Press. https://nap.nationalacademies.org/catalog/10534/immunization-safety-review-sv40-contamination-of-polio-vaccine-and-cancer.

8   Ibid.

9   Ratner, H. Illinois Medical Journal. (1960). Volume 118, Issue 2. Retrieved from https://archive.org/details/sim_illinois-medical-journal_1960-08_118_2/page/84/mode/2up.

10   National Security Zone, Medill School of Journalism, Northwestern University. (n.d.). "What the 1916 NYC Polio Epidemic Can Tell Us About COVID-19." Retrieved from https://nationalsecurityzone.medill.northwestern.edu/covidanalyzer/news/what-the-1916-nyc-polio-epidemic-can-tell-us-about-covid-19/.

11   National Institute of Food and Agriculture (NIFA), US Department of Agriculture. (n.d.). "Pesticide Trends." Retrieved from https://www.nifa.usda.gov/sites/default/files/resources/Pesticide%20Trends.pdf.

12   Wyatt, HV. "The 1916 New York City Epidemic of Poliomyelitis: Where did the Virus Come From?" *The Open Vaccine Journal*, 2011, 4, 13–17 https://benthamopen.com/contents/pdf/TOVACJ/TOVACJ-4-13.pdf.

13   Ibid.

14   West, J. "Pesticides and Polio." 2014. https://harvoa.org/polio/overview.htm

15   Carson, R. (2002). *Silent Spring*. Houghton Mifflin Harcourt. https://www.amazon.com/Silent-Spring-Rachel-Carson/dp/0618249060

16   Lea A. Cupul-Uicab. "Exposure to DDT from indoor residual spraying and biomarkers of inflammation among reproductive-aged women from South Africa," *Environmental Research*, Volume 191, 2020, https://doi.org /10.1016/j.envres.2020.110088.

17   Hotez, P. J., & Ferris, M. T. (2019). "The broad spectrum of poliovirus infection: From acute paralytic disease to chronic sequelae." *Clinical Microbiology Reviews*, 32(4), e00038–19. https://doi.org/10.1128/CMR.00038–19.

18   US Environmental Protection Agency (EPA). (2003). Health assessment document for DDT. EPA/600/8–83/021F. Retrieved from https://semspub. epa.gov/work/03/2087981.pdf.

19   Miller, G. W., & Jones, D. P. (2014). "The role of environmental factors in neurodegenerative diseases." Current Environmental Health Reports, 1(2), 123–132. https://doi.org/10.1007/s40572–014-0012–1.

20   Trevelyan, B. "The Spatial Dynamics of Poliomyelitis in the United States: From Epidemic Emergence to Vaccine-Induced Retreat, 1910–1971." Ann Assoc Am Geogr. 2005 Jun;95(2):269–293. doi: 10.1111/j.1467–8306. 2005.00460.x.

21   Murray, J. A. "Century of Tuberculosis," *American Journal of Respiratory and Critical Care Medicine*,Vol.169,N.11, pp.1181–1186},2004 doi: 10.1164/ rccm.200402–140OE.

22   Goldman AS, Schmalstieg EJ, Dreyer CF, Schmalstieg FC Jr, Goldman DA. "Franklin Delano Roosevelt's (FDR's) (1882–1945) 1921 neurological disease revisited; the most likely diagnosis remains Guillain-Barré syndrome." *J Med Biogr.* 2016 Nov;24(4):452–459. doi: 10.1177/0967772015605738.

23   Our World in Data. (n.d.). Polio. Retrieved from https://ourworldindata .org/polio.

24   West, J. "Pesticides and Polio." 2014. https://harvoa.org/polio/overview.htm.

25   Centers for Disease Control and Prevention (CDC). (2019). Poliomyelitis. In Epidemiology and Prevention of Vaccine-Preventable Diseases (The Pink Book) (13th ed.). Retrieved from https://stacks.cdc.gov/view/cdc/74158.

26   Centers for Disease Control and Prevention (CDC). (n.d.). Chapter 18: Poliomyelitis. In Epidemiology and Prevention of Vaccine-Preventable Diseases (The Pink Book). Retrieved from https://www.cdc.gov/pinkbook /hcp/table-of-contents/chapter-18-poliomyelitis.html#:~:text=Inactivated %20poliovirus%20(IPV)%20vaccine%20was,(tOPV)%20vaccine%20 in%201963.

27   Global Polio Eradication Initiative. (n.d.). Inactivated Polio Vaccine (IPV). Retrieved from https://polioeradication.org/about-polio/the-vaccines/ipv/.

28   Fine, P. E., & Carneiro, I. A. (2011). "Transmissibility and fading immunity following oral poliovirus vaccine." *The Lancet Infectious Diseases*, 11(5), 345–350.

29   Saloni Dattani, et al. (2022) "Polio" Published online at OurWorldinData. org. Retrieved from: https://ourworldindata.org/grapher/cases-of-paralytic -polio-from-wild-vs-vaccine-derived-viruses?time=2015..latest [Online Resource].

30   Centers for Disease Control and Prevention (CDC). (n.d.). Vaccinate with Confidence. Retrieved from https://www.cdc.gov/vaccines/covid-19/vacci-nate-with-confidence.html.

Chapter 4

1   Anderson, M. L. "The Effect of Influenza Vaccination for the Elderly on Hospitalization and Mortality: An Observational Study with a Regression Discontinuity Design." *Ann Intern Med*. 2020 Apr 7;172(7):445–452. doi: 10.7326/M19-3075.

2   Centers for Disease Control and Prevention. "Influenza (Flu)." CDC, www .cdc.gov/flu/.

3   Centers for Disease Control and Prevention. "FluView: Weekly Influenza Surveillance Report, Week 17, 2025." CDC, www.cdc.gov/fluview/surveillance /2025-week-17.html.

4   Centers for Disease Control and Prevention. "Estimated Flu Disease Burden, 2024–2025." CDC, www.cdc.gov/flu-burden/php/data-vis/2024–2025.html.

5   Centers for Disease Control and Prevention. "CDC's Advisory Committee on Immunization Concludes Meeting with Joint Statement." CDC Newsroom, 26 June 2025, www.cdc.gov/media/releases/2025/s0626-acip-meeting.html.

6   Centers for Disease Control and Prevention. "Adjuvanted Flu Vaccine." CDC, www.cdc.gov/flu/vaccine-types/adjuvant.html.

7   Branswell, Helen. "CDC Vaccine Promotions Under Scrutiny as RFK Jr. Pushes for Informed Consent." STAT, 20 Feb. 2025, www.statnews .com/2025/02/20/cdc-vaccine-promotions-rfk-jr-informed-consent/.

8   Lee, J. K. H. "High-dose influenza vaccine in older adults by age and seasonal characteristics: Systematic review and meta-analysis update." *Vaccine X*. 2023 Jun 5;14:100327. doi: 10.1016/j.jvacx.2023.100327

9   Simonsen L, Reichert TA, Viboud C, Blackwelder WC, Taylor RJ, Miller MA. "Impact of influenza vaccination on seasonal mortality in the US elderly population." *Arch Intern Med*. 2005 Feb 14;165(3):265–72. doi: 10.1001/archinte.165.3.265.

10 Shrestha, N. et al. "Effectiveness of the Influenza Vaccine During the 2024–2025 Respiratory Viral Season," *medRxiv* 2025.01.30.25321421; doi: https: //doi.org/10.1101/2025.01.30.25321421.

11 Centers for Disease Control and Prevention. "Preliminary Estimated Flu Disease Burden 2024–2025 Flu Season." CDC, 8 May 2025, www.cdc.gov /flu-burden/php/data-vis/2024–2025.html.

12 Bystrianyk, Roman. "Did Vaccines Reduce Flu and Pneumonia?" Roman Bystrianyk on Substack, 16 Apr. 2025, romanbystrianyk.substack.com/p /did-vaccines-reduce-flu-and-pneumonia.

13 Bi, Q. "US Flu Vaccine Effectiveness Network Investigators. Reduced Effectiveness of Repeat Influenza Vaccination: Distinguishing Among Within-Season Waning, Recent Clinical Infection, and Subclinical Infection." *J Infect Dis.* 2024 Dec 16;230(6):1309–1318. doi: 10.1093/infdis/jiae220.

14 Food and Drug Administration. "Vaccines and Related Biological Products Advisory Committee Meeting: Influenza Virus Vaccine Composition for the 2015–2016 Season." FDA, 4 Mar. 2015, www.fda.gov/media/94583/download.

15 Wolff G. G. "Influenza vaccination and respiratory virus interference among Department of Defense personnel during the 2017–2018 influenza season." *Vaccine.* 2020 Jan 10;38(2):350–354. doi: 10.1016/j.vaccine.2019.10.005.

16 Mishra, Manas. "Moderna Pulls Application for COVID-Flu Combination Shot." Reuters, 21 May 2025, www.reuters.com/business/healthcare-pharmaceuticals/moderna-withdraws-application-covid-flu-combination-vaccine-2025-05-21/.

17 Ibid.

Chapter 5

1 Davis, E. Y. (May 2023). Why you should never, ever take an mRNA vaccine. https://realhealthflash.substack.com/p/why-you-should-never-ever-take-an.

2 Prasad V., Makary M. A. "An evidence-based approach to Covid-19 vaccination." *N Engl J Med.* 2025. doi: 10.1056/NEJMsb2506929 https://www.nejm.org/doi/full/10.1056/NEJMsb2506929.

3 Ibid.

4 Makary, M. (2025, April 30). Quoted in Fox News. "FDA approves updated COVID-19 vaccines: What to know about the new shots." Retrieved from https://www.foxnews.com/health/fda-approves-updated-covid-19-vaccines-what-know-new-shots.

5   Prasad V., Makary M. A. "An evidence-based approach to Covid-19 vaccination."

6   Ibid.

7   Adams M. L., Katz D. L., Grandpre J. "Population-based estimates of chronic conditions affecting risk for complications from coronavirus disease, United States." *Emerg Infect Dis* 2020;26:1831–1833. https://pubmed.ncbi.nlm.nih.gov/32324118/.

8   "Benefits of Getting a COVID-19 Vaccine." Centers for Disease Control and Prevention, www.cdc.gov/covid/vaccines/benefits.html. Accessed 6 June 2025.

9   Polack, F. P., et al. (2020). Safety and efficacy of the BNT162b2 mRNA Covid-19 vaccine." *New England Journal of Medicine*, 383(27), 2603–2615. doi:10.1056/NEJMoa2034577.

10 Baden, L. R., et al. (2021). "Efficacy and safety of the mRNA-1273 SARS-CoV-2 vaccine." *New England Journal of Medicine*, 384(5), 403–416. doi:10.1056/NEJMoa2035389.

11 Shrestha N. K., et al. "Effectiveness of the 2023–2024 Formulation of the COVID-19 Messenger RNA Vaccine." *Clin Infect Dis.* 2024 Aug 16;79(2):405–411. doi: 10.1093/cid/ciae132. https://pubmed.ncbi.nlm.nih.gov/38465901/.

12 Ioannou, G. N., et al. (2022). "COVID-19 vaccination effectiveness against infection or death in a national US health care system: A target trial emulation study." *Annals of Internal Medicine*, 175(3), 352–361. https://doi.org/10.7326/M21–3256[](https://pubmed.ncbi.nlm.nih.gov/34280332/).

13 Nakatani, E., Morioka, H., Kikuchi, T., & Fukushima, M. (2024). "Behavioral and health outcomes of mRNA COVID-19 vaccination: A case-control study in Japanese small and medium-sized enterprises." *Cureus*, 16(12), e75652. https://doi.org/10.7759/cureus.75652[](https://pubmed.ncbi.nlm.nih.gov/39803093/).

14   Eythorsson, E., Runolfsdottir, H. L., Ingvarsson, R. F., Sigurdsson, M. I., & Palsson, R. (2022). "Rate of SARS-CoV-2 reinfection during an Omicron wave in Iceland." *JAMA Network Open*, 5(8), e2225320. https://doi.org /10.1001/jamanetworkopen.2022.25320[](https://palexander.substack.com /p/eythorsson-et-al-rate-of-sars-cov).

15   Chemaitelly, H., et al. (2022). "Protection against reinfection with the Omicron BA.2.75 subvariant." *The New England Journal of Medicine*, 388(7), 665–667.   https://doi.org/10.1056/NEJMc2214114[](https://pubmed.ncbi .nlm.nih.gov/38591115/).

16   Shrestha N. K., et al. "Effectiveness of the 2023–2024 Formulation of the COVID-19 Messenger RNA Vaccine."

17   Feldstein, L. R., Griggs, E., Levintow, S., Taylor, C. A., Haggard, R., Rowley, E., . . . Feldstein, L. R. (2023). "Waning effectiveness of mRNA COVID-19 vaccines in children aged 5–11 years in the United States: A test-negative case-control study." *The Lancet Regional Health—Americas, 27,* 100614. https://doi.org/10.1016/j.lana.2023.100614.

18   Irrgang, P. et al. (2023). "Class switch toward noninflammatory, spike-specific IgG4 antibodies after repeated SARS-CoV-2 mRNA vaccination." *Science Immunology,* 8(79), eade2798. https://doi.org/10.1126/sciimmunol .ade2798.

19   Bergwerk, M. (2021). "COVID-19 breakthrough infections in vaccinated health care workers." *New England Journal of Medicine*, 385(16), 1474–1484. https://doi.org/10.1056/NEJMoa2109072.

20   Sun, L. H. (2025, April 30). "RFK Jr. will order placebo testing for new vaccines, alarming health experts." *The Washington Post.* https://www.washing tonpost.com/health/2025/04/30/rfk-jr-vaccine-testing/.

21   ModernaTX, Inc. "A Study of mRNA-1283.222 Injection Compared with mRNA-1273.222 Injection in Participants ≥12 Years of Age to Prevent COVID-19 (NextCOVE)." ClinicalTrials.gov, 18 Apr. 2023, classic.clinical trials.gov/ct2/show/NCT05815498. Accessed 6 June 2025.

22 Moderna, Inc. (2024, March 26). "Moderna achieves positive interim results from Phase 3 trial of next-generation COVID-19 vaccine." Moderna News Releases. https://investors.modernatx.com/news/news-details/2024 /Moderna-Achieves-Positive-Interim-Results-from-Phase-3-Trial-of-Next -Generation-COVID-19-Vaccine/default.aspx.

23 US Food and Drug Administration. (2023, August). "Pfizer-BioNTech COVID-19 vaccine (2023–2024 Formula)" [Package insert]. https://www .fda.gov/media/159897/download.

24 Schaffer et al. "Effect of the 2022 COVID-19 booster vaccination campaign in people aged 50 years in England." *Vaccine.* V 59. June 2025 https://www .sciencedirect.com/science/article/pii/S0264410X25005547.

25 US Food and Drug Administration. (2023, August). "Moderna COVID-19 vaccine (2023–2024 Formula)" [Package insert]. https://www.fda.gov/media /151707/download.

26 *Pfizer/BioNTech's COVID-19 modRNA Vaccines: Dangerous Genetic Mechanism of Action, Released before Sufficient Preclinical Testing, The Pfizer Papers: Pfizer's Crimes Against Humanity.* Naomi Wolf, Editor. Oct 2024. Skyhorse Publishing. NY, NY.

27 Rogers, C., Thorp, J., Cosgrove, K., & McCullough, P. (2024). "COVID-19 vaccines: A risk factor for cerebral thrombotic syndromes." *International Journal of Innovative Research in Medical Science*, 9(11), 621–627. https://doi .org/10.23958/ijirms/vol09-i11/1982

28 Saji, T., & Matsuzaki, T. (2024). "Myocarditis and pericarditis following mRNA COVID-19 vaccination in Japanese pediatric cases." *Circulation Journal.* Advance online publication. https://www.jstage.jst.go.jp/article/circj /advpub/0/advpub_CJ-24–0506/_article.

29 Hulscher, N., Hodkinson, R., Makis, W., McCullough, P. A., & Malhotra, A. (2024). "A systematic review of autopsy findings in deaths after COVID-19 vaccination." *Cureus*, 16(1), e52365. https://doi.org/10.7759/cureus.52365.

30 https://www.fda.gov/media/186738/download?attachment=&utm_source =substack&utm_medium=email.

31 https://www.opastpublishers.com/open-access-articles/excess-cardio pulmonary-arrest-and-mortality-after-covid19-vaccination-in-king-county -washington.pdf J Emerg Med OA, 2(1), 01–11.

32 Retsef, Levi, Fahad Mansuri, Melissa M. Jordan, Joseph A. Ladapo. "Twelve-Month All-Cause Mortality after Initial COVID-19 Vaccination with Pfizer-BioNTech or mRNA-1273 among Adults Living in Florida," MedRxiv, https://doi.org/10.1101/2025.04.25.25326460.

33 https://publichealthpolicyjournal.com/a-systematic-review-of-autopsy-findings -in-deaths-after-covid-19-vaccination/.

34 Kakeya H., Nitta T., Kamijima Y., Miyazawa T. "Significant Increase in Excess Deaths after Repeated COVID-19 Vaccination in Japan." *JMA J.* 2025;8(2):584–586 https://www.jmaj.jp/detail.php?id=10.31662%2Fjmaj.2024 –0298.

35 Faksova et al., Vaccine, 2024;42(9):2200–2211. doi:10.1016/j.vaccine.2024.01 .100 https://www.sciencedirect.com/science/article/pii/S0264410X24001270.

36 Karimi et al., *Int J Prev Med*, 2025;16:14. doi:10.4103/ijpvm.ijpvm_260 _24, https://journals.lww.com/ijom/fulltext/2025/03210/covid_19_vaccination _and_cardiovascular_events_a.6.aspx.

37 Ibid.

38 Faksova, K., et al. "COVID-19 Vaccines and Adverse Events of Special Interest: A Multinational Global Vaccine Data Network (GVDN) Cohort Study of 99 Million Vaccinated Individuals." *Vaccine*, vol. 42, no. 9, 2024, pp. 2200–2211. https://doi.org/10.1016/j.vaccine.2024.01.100.

39 Humanspective. (2025, February 4). Stunning. Pfizer like plasmids found in a cancer biopsy of someone that had 4 x Pfizer's vaccine. X. https://x.com /Humanspective/status/1886631440932343945.

40 Aldén, M., et al. (2022). "Intracellular Reverse Transcription of Pfizer BioNTech COVID-19 mRNA Vaccine BNT162b2 In Vitro in Human Liver Cell Line." *Current Issues in Molecular Biology*, 44(3), 1115–1126. https://doi.org/10.3390/cimb44030073[](https://pubmed.ncbi.nlm.nih .gov/35723296/).

41 Angueira, R. V., & Perea Bustos, Y. (2023). "SARS-CoV-2 vaccination and the multi-hit hypothesis of oncogenesis." *Cureus*, 15(12), Article e50703. https://doi.org/10.7759/cureus.50703.

42 Erdoğdu, B., et al. (2024). "Metabolomic profiling of leukemic hemato-poiesis: Effects of BNT162b2 mRNA COVID-19 vaccine administration." Current Cancer Drug Targets. Advance online publication. https://www .eurekaselect.com/article/148704.

43 Abue, M., et al. (2025). "Repeated COVID-19 Vaccination as a Poor Prognostic Factor in Pancreatic Cancer: A Retrospective, Single-Center Cohort Study." *Cancers*, 17(12), 2006. https://doi.org/10.3390/cancers17122006.

44 Bhattacharjee, B., and A. Iwasaki. "Immune Markers of Post-Vaccination Syndrome Indicate Future Research Directions." *Yale News*, 25 Feb. 2025. https://news.yale.edu/2025/02/25/immune-markers-post-vaccination -syndrome-indicate-future-research-directions.

45 Ota, K., et al. (2025). "Expression of SARS-CoV-2 spike protein in cerebral arteries: Implications for hemorrhagic stroke post-mRNA vaccination." *Journal of Clinical Neuroscience*, 136, 111223. https://doi.org/10.1016/j.jocn .2025.111223.

46 Rasmussen Reports. (2025, May 29). "COVID-19: 51% suspect heart damage from vaccine." Rasmussen Reports. https://www.rasmussenreports.com /public_content/lifestyle/covid_19/covid_19_51_suspect_heart_damage_from _vaccine?utm_source=substack&utm_medium=email.

47 Mead, M. N., Rose, J., Makis, W., Milhoan, K., Hulscher, N., & McCullough, P. A. (2025). "Landmark analysis finds COVID-19 vaccine myocarditis is more common and severe than SARS-CoV-2 infection

myocarditis." *International Journal of Cardiovascular Research & Innovation.* https://doi.org/10.61577/ijcri.2025.100001.

48 Buergin N, et al. "Sex-specific differences in myocardial injury incidence after COVID-19 mRNA-1273 booster vaccination." *Eur J Heart Fail.* 2023 Oct;25(10):1871–1881. doi: 10.1002/ejhf.2978.

49 Nakamura, M., & Nakamura, K. (2025). "Cardiac imaging findings after SARS-CoV-2 infection and vaccination in a large cohort." *Circulation Journal,* 89(1), Article CJ-24–0506. https://doi.org/10.1253/circj.CJ-24–0506.

50 Mead, M. N., Rose, J., Makis, W., Milhoan, K., Hulscher, N., & McCullough, P. A. (2023). "Myocarditis after SARS-CoV-2 infection and COVID-19 vaccination: Epidemiology, outcomes, and new perspectives." *INTERNATIONAL JOURNAL OF CARDIOVASCULAR RESEARCH & INNOVATION* Jan-Mar 2025, VOL. 3, ISSUE 1, pp. 1–43 https://cardiovascular-research-and-innovation.reseaprojournals.com/article/myocarditis-after-sars-cov-2-infection-and-covid-19-vaccination-epidemiology-outcomes-and-new-perspectives.

51 Kim, J. H., Lee, S. Y., & Park, H. J. (2023). "Cardiac imaging findings after SARS-CoV-2 infection and vaccination in a large cohort." *Journal of Cardiovascular Imaging,* 35(2), 98–107. https://doi.org/10.3346/jci.2023.35.2.98.

52 Szebeni J. "Expanded Spectrum and Increased Incidence of Adverse Events Linked to COVID-19 Genetic Vaccines: New Concepts on Prophylactic Immuno-Gene Therapy, Iatrogenic Orphan Disease, and Platform-Inherent Challenges." *Pharmaceutics.* 2025; 17(4):450. https://doi.org/10.3390/pharmaceutics17040450.

53 Cheng, K.-L., and M.-S. Tsai. "Long-Term Thyroid Outcomes After COVID-19 Vaccination: A Cohort Study of 2,333,496 Patients from the TriNetX Network." *Journal of Clinical Endocrinology & Metabolism,* vol. 110, no. 7, 2025, Article dgaf064. https://doi.org/10.1210/clinem/dgaf064.

54   Thorp, J., Drew Pinsky and Peter McCullough. (2025) "Association between COVID-19 Vaccination and Neuropsychiatric Conditions" Preprints. https://doi.org/10.20944/preprints202504.1099.v1.

55   Pfizer. (2023, December 14). Pfizer completes acquisition of Seagen [Press release]. https://www.pfizer.com/news/press-release/press-release-detail/pfizer-completes-acquisition-seagen.

Chapter 6

1   Bhattacharya, J., & Bridgen, A. (2024, August 7). "Dr. Jay Bhattacharya and Andrew Bridgen - FreeNZ "[Video]. Rumble. https://rumble.com/v59emm4-dr-jay-bhattacharya-and-andrew-bridgen-freenz.html.

2   https://apnews.com/article/fact-check-covid-vaccines-gene-therapy-806280914802.

3   https://www.pfizer.com/news/behind-the-science/unlocking-power-our-bodys-protein-factory#:

4   Vanden Bossche, Geert, and Robert Rennebohm. 2023. *The Inescapable Immune Escape Pandemic*. Dallas, TX: Pierucci Publishing.

5   Shrestha N. K., Burke P. C., Nowacki A. S., Gordon S. M. "Effectiveness of the 2023–2024 Formulation of the COVID-19 Messenger RNA Vaccine." *Clin Infect Dis.* 2024 Aug 16;79(2):405–411. doi: 10.1093/cid/ciae132. https://pubmed.ncbi.nlm.nih.gov/38465901/.

6   https://www.pfizer.com/science/innovation/mrna-technology.

7   Fraiman, J. (2022). "Serious adverse events of special interest following mRNA COVID-19 vaccination in randomized trials in adults." *Vaccine*, 40(26), 3537–3541. https://doi.org/10.1016/j.vaccine.2022.02.037.

8   Brogna, C. "Detection of recombinant Spike protein in the blood of individuals vaccinated against SARS-CoV-2: Possible molecular mechanisms." 31 August 2023 https://doi.org/10.1002/prca.202300048.

9   Bhattacharjee, B., and A. Iwasaki. "Immune Markers of Post-Vaccination Syndrome Indicate Future Research Directions." *Yale News*, 25 Feb. 2025. https://news.yale.edu/2025/02/25/immune-markers-post-vaccination -syndrome-indicate-future-research-directions.

10 McCullough, P. (2023). "Clinical rationale for SARS-CoV-2 base spike protein detoxification in post-COVID-19 and vaccine injury syndromes." *Journal of American Physicians and Surgeons*, 28(3), 90–94. https://jpands .org/vol28no3/mccullough.pdf.

11 @MDBreathe. (2025, May 19). X Post. Presents data on spike protein IgG antibody levels.

12 McCullough, P. (2023). "Clinical rationale for SARS-CoV-2 base spike protein detoxification."

13 Independent Medical Alliance (IMA). (2023, May 9). I-PREVENT: Vaccine Injury Protocol. https://imahealth.org/protocol/i-prevent-vaccine-injury/.

14 Pfizer Inc. The Facts. Retrieved from https://www.pfizer.com/about /responsibility/misinformation?utm_source=substack&utm_medium=email.

15 Markov, P.V., Ghafari, M., Beer, M. et al. "The evolution of SARS-CoV-2." *Nat Rev Microbiol* 21, 361–379 (2023). https://doi.org/10.1038 /s41579–023-00878–2.

16 Hulscher, N. "Pfizer Busted Using Irrelevant Study to Deny Genome Integration Risks from Their mRNA Injections." Retrieved from https: //www.thefocalpoints.com/p/breaking-pfizer-busted-using-irrelevant?r =o3im2&utm_campaign=post&utm_medium=web&showWelcomeOnShare =false.

17 https://inmodia.de/en/services/detection-of-spike-protein/.

18 Hulscher, N. "BREAKING—Reverse Transcription, Abnormal Gene Expression Detected in Patients After mRNA Vaccination." Retrieved from https://www.thefocalpoints.com/p/breaking-reverse-transcription-cancer ?utm_source=substack&utm_medium=email.

19 Kyriakopoulos, A. M., & McCullough, P. A. (2022). "Potential mechanisms for human genome integration of genetic code from SARS-CoV-2 mRNA vaccination: Implications for disease." *Journal of Clinical Immunology and Immunotherapy*, 8(1), 1–8. https://doi.org/10.36648/2471–256X.8.1.92500.

20 Aldén M., Olofsson Falla F., Yang D., Barghouth M., Luan C., Rasmussen M., De Marinis Y. "Intracellular Reverse Transcription of Pfizer BioNTech COVID-19 mRNA Vaccine BNT162b2 In Vitro in Human Liver Cell Line." *Current Issues in Molecular Biology*. 2022; 44(3):1115–1126. https://doi.org/10.3390/cimb44030073.

21 https://www.nature.com/articles/s41586–023-06800–3.

22 Mulroney, T. E., Pöyry, T., Yam-Puc, J. C., et al. (2023). "N1-methylpseudouridylation of mRNA causes +1 ribosomal frameshifting." *Nature*, 621(7980), 372–379. https://doi.org/10.1038/s41586–023-06800–3[](https://www.nature.com/articles/s41586–023-06800–3).

23 Ibid.

24 Adl-Tabatabai, Sean. "New NIH Director Warns 'Dangerous mRNA Jabs' Are Causing Millions to Die." *The People's Voice,* May 14, 2025. https://thepeoplesvoice.tv/new-nih-director-warns-dangerous-mrna-jabs-are-causing-millions-to-die/.

25 Ibid.

26 McKernan, K. et al. 2023. "Sequencing of Bivalent Moderna and Pfizer Mrna Vaccines Reveals Nanogram to Microgram Quantities of Expression Vector Dsdna Per Dose." OSF Preprints. April 10. doi:10.31219/osf.io/b9t7m.

27 Speicher, David & Rose, Jessica & Gutschi, Luz & Wiseman, David & McKernan, Kevin. (2023)., "DNA fragments detected in COVID-19 vaccines in Canada. DNA fragments detected in monovalent and bivalent."

28 Chartier, N., & Horwood, M. (2023, October 19). "EXCLUSIVE: Health Canada Confirms Undisclosed Presence of DNA Sequence in Pfizer Shot." *The Epoch Times.* https://www.theepochtimes.com/world/exclusive

-health-canada-confirms-undisclosed-presence-of-dna-sequence-in-pfizer -shot-5513277.

29   McKernan, K. "Sequencing of Bivalent Moderna and Pfizer Mrna Vaccines Reveals Nanogram to Microgram Quantities of Expression Vector Dsdna Per Dose."

30   Ibid.

31   Ibid.

32   Ibid.

33   Mörtenhuber, W. (2022, August 31). "Re: Covid-19 vaccines and treatments: we must have raw data, now." *The BMJ*, 378, o1731. https://www .bmj.com/content/378/bmj.o1731/rr-2.

34   Flowers, C., et al. War Room/*DailyClout* Pfizer Documents Investigators. (2023, October 6). "Report 86: Pfizer's Clinical Trial 'Process 2' COVID Vaccine Recipients Suffered 2.4X the Adverse Events of Placebo Recipients; 'Process 2' Vials Were Contaminated with DNA Plasmids." *DailyClout*. https://daily clout.io/pfizer-process-2-vaccine-had-2–4-times-adverse-events/[](https: //dailyclout.io/pfizer-process-2-vaccine-had-2–4-times-adverse-events/).

35   US Food and Drug Administration. (2020). Emergency Use Authorization (EUA) Letter: Pfizer-BioNTech COVID-19 Vaccine. Retrieved from https://www.fda.gov/emergency-preparedness-and-response/mcm-legal -regulatory-and-policy-framework/emergency-use-authorization.

36   Speicher, David & Rose, Jessica & Gutschi, Luz & Wiseman, David & McKernan, Kevin. (2023). "DNA fragments detected in COVID-19 vaccines in Canada. DNA fragments detected in monovalent and bivalent."

37   Ledford, H. (2023, December 6). "mRNA vaccines may make unintended proteins, but there's no evidence of harm." *Nature*. https://www.nature.com /articles/d41586–023-03859-w.

38 Kitonsa, J. et al. "Safety and Immunogenicity of a Modified Self-Amplifying Ribonucleic Acid (saRNA) Vaccine Encoding SARS-CoV-2 Spike Glycoprotein in SARS-CoV-2 Seronegative and Seropositive Ugandan Individuals." *Vaccines*, *13*(6), 553. 2025. https://doi.org/10.3390/vaccines13060553.

39 Ibid.

40 BARDA is a US government agency within the Department of Health and Human Services (HHS), specifically under the Office of the Assistant Secretary for Preparedness and Response (ASPR). Established in 2006 through the Pandemic and All-Hazards Preparedness Act, BARDA's mission is to develop and procure *medical countermeasures* (e.g., vaccines, therapeutics, diagnostics) to protect against public health threats, including pandemics, bioterrorism, chemical, biological, radiological, and nuclear (CBRN) incidents.

41 Neale, T. (2023, July 29). "Covid vaccine: What uptake of new shots could look like." https://www.cnbc.com/2023/07/29/covid-vaccine-what-uptake-of-new-shots-could-look-like.html.

42 Constantino, A. (2023, October 26). "Pfizer's combination Covid, flu vaccine shows positive trial data." CNBC. https://www.cnbc.com/2023/10/26/pfizer-combination-covid-flu-vaccine-shows-positive-trial-data.html.

43 Tucker, J. A. (2023, August 28). "Delights of the Pfizer/Moderna catfight." Brownstone Institute. https://brownstone.org/articles/delights-of-the-pfizer-moderna-catfight/.

44 Garde, D. (2016, September 13). "Ego, ambition, and turmoil: Inside one of biotech's most secretive startups." *STAT News*. https://www.statnews.com/2016/09/13/moderna-therapeutics-biotech-mrna/.

45 Dolgin, E. (2024). "mRNA vaccines: Hope beneath the hype." *Nature Reviews Drug Discovery*, 23(2), 89–94. https://doi.org/10.1038/s41573-023-00859-3.

46 https://www.ncbi.nlm.nih.gov/pmc/articles/PMC7794803/.

47   https://doi.org/10.1038/s41578–021-00358–0.

48   https://www.frontiersin.org/articles/10.3389/fimmu.2020.603039/full.

49   https://www.ahajournals.org/doi/10.1161/STROKEAHA.122.040430.

50   https://bmjopen.bmj.com/content/13/6/e065687.

51   https://jamanetwork.com/journals/jama/fullarticle/2788346.

52   https://www.westernstandard.news/business/pfizer-s-own-study-finds-nano
     particles-in-covid-vaccines-enter-organs/article_5b3955f6-d146–11ec-a272
     -cf3264db392b.html.

53   Shrestha, N. K., et al. "Risk of coronavirus disease 2019 (COVID-19) acqui-
     sition for healthcare workers by vaccination status and the evolving risk with
     the delta and omicron variants."

54   Shrestha, N. K., et al. (2022). "Coronavirus disease 2019 vaccine boosting in
     previously infected or vaccinated individuals." medRxiv. https://doi.org/10
     .1101/2022.12.17.22283625.

Chapter 7

1   Centers for Disease Control and Prevention. (2024). About shingles (herpes
     zoster). US Department of Health and Human Services. https://www.cdc
     .gov/shingles/about/.

2   US Food and Drug Administration. (2017). Shingrix (Zoster Vaccine
     Recombinant, Adjuvanted): Package insert. US Department of Health and
     Human Services. https://www.fda.gov/media/108597/download.

3   Zerbo O., Bartlett J., Fireman B., et al. "Recombinant Zoster Vaccination
     and Risk of Postherpetic Neuralgia or Zoster Ophthalmicus." *JAMA Netw
     Open*. 2025;8(6):e2514615. doi:10.1001/jamanetworkopen.2025.14615.

4   Ibid.

5   Ibid.

Chapter 8

1   Bonten, M. et al· "Polysaccharide Conjugate Vaccine against Pneumococcal Pneumonia in Adults" Authors: Randomized Controlled Trial, *N Engl J Med.* 2015 Mar 19;372(12):1114–25. doi: 10.1056/NEJMoa1408544. https://www.nejm.org/doi/full/10.1056/NEJMoa1408544.

2   Tsaban, G., & Ben-Shimol, S. (2017). "Indirect (herd) protection, following pneumococcal conjugated vaccines introduction: A systematic review of the literature." *Vaccine*, 35(22), 2882–2891. https://doi.org/10.1016/j.vaccine.2017.04.032[](https://pmc.ncbi.nlm.nih.gov/articles/PMC8903918/).

3   US Food and Drug Administration. (2024). "Capvaxive: 21-valent pneumococcal conjugate vaccine." US Department of Health and Human Services. https://www.fda.gov/vaccines-blood-biologics/capvaxive.

4   US Food and Drug Administration. (2017). Prevnar 13 (pneumococcal 13-valent conjugate vaccine): Package insert. US Department of Health and Human Services. https://www.fda.gov/media/80547/download?attachment.

5   US Food and Drug Administration. (2021). Prevnar 20 (Pneumococcal 20-valent Conjugate Vaccine): Package insert. US Department of Health and Human Services. https://www.fda.gov/media/149987/download?attachment.

6   US Food and Drug Administration. (2020). Pneumovax 23 (Pneumococcal Vaccine Polyvalent): Package insert. US Department of Health and Human Services. https://www.fda.gov/media/77395/download.

Chapter 9

1   Centers for Disease Control and Prevention. (2024). RSV Surveillance & Research. Retrieved from https://www.cdc.gov/rsv/php/surveillance/index.html.

2   Ibid.

3   US Food and Drug Administration. (2023). Abrysvo (Respiratory Syncytial Virus Vaccine): Package insert. US Department of Health and Human Services. https://www.fda.gov/media/168889/download.

4   Ison, M. G., Papi, A., Athan, E., Feldman, R. G., Langley, J. M., Lee, D.-G., . . . & Esser, M. T. (2024). "Safety and immunogenicity of a bivalent RSV prefusion F vaccine in older adults." *JAMA Network Open, 7*(8), e2428058. https://doi.org/10.1001/jamanetworkopen.2024.28058.

5   US Food and Drug Administration. (2023). Arexvy (Respiratory Syncytial Virus Vaccine, Adjuvanted): Package insert. US Department of Health and Human Services. https://www.fda.gov/files/vaccines%2C%20blood%20%26%20biologics/published/Package-Insert-AREXVY.pdf.

6   US Food and Drug Administration. (2024). mRESVIA (Respiratory Syncytial Virus Vaccine, mRNA): Package insert. US Department of Health and Human Services. https://www.fda.gov/media/179005/download.

7   US Food and Drug Administration. (2024). "FDA requires Guillain-Barré Syndrome (GBS) warning in prescribing information for RSV vaccines Abrysvo and Arexvy." US Department of Health and Human Services. https://www.fda.gov/vaccines-blood-biologics/safety-availability-biologics/fda-requires-guillain-barre-syndrome-gbs-warning-prescribing-information-rsv-vaccines-abrysvo-and.

8   US Food and Drug Administration. (2023). Abrysvo (Respiratory Syncytial Virus Vaccine): Package insert. US Department of Health and Human Services. https://www.fda.gov/media/168889/download.

9   Centers for Disease Control and Prevention. (2023). GRADE: Pfizer Bivalent RSVpreF vaccine for adults. US Department of Health and Human Services. https://www.cdc.gov/acip/grade/Pfizer-Bivalent-RSVpreF-adults.html.

10 US Food and Drug Administration. (2023). Arexvy (Respiratory Syncytial Virus Vaccine, Adjuvanted): Package insert. US Department of Health and Human Services. https://www.fda.gov/files/vaccines%2C%20blood%26biologics/published/Package-Insert-AREXVY.pdf.

Chapter 10

1   Centers for Disease Control and Prevention (CDC). "Tetanus." Accessed May 31, 2025. https://www.cdc.gov/tetanus/index.html.

2   World Health Organization (WHO). "Tetanus vaccines: WHO position paper – February 2017." Weekly Epidemiological Record, 92 (2017): 53–76.

3   US Food and Drug Administration (FDA). "Vaccines Licensed for Use in the United States." Accessed May 31, 2025. https://www.fda.gov /vaccines-blood-biologics/vaccines/vaccines-licensed-use-united-states.

4   Geier, D.A., and Geier, M.R. "A review of the vaccine adverse event reporting system database." Expert Opinion on Drug Safety, 6(6) (2007): 691–698.

5   Ibid.

6   Ibid.

7   Institute of Medicine (US) Vaccine Safety Committee; Stratton KR, Howe CJ, Johnston RB Jr., editors. "Adverse Events Associated with Childhood Vaccines: Evidence Bearing on Causality." Washington (DC): National Academies Press (US); 1994. 5, Diphtheria and Tetanus Toxoids. https: //www.ncbi.nlm.nih.gov/books/NBK236292/.

8   US Food and Drug Administration. (2019). TDVAX (Tetanus and Diphtheria Toxoids Adsorbed): Package insert. US Department of Health and Human Services. https://www.fda.gov/media/76430/download.

9   Geier, D. A., & Geier, M. R. (2004). "A review of the Vaccine Adverse Event Reporting System database." Expert Opinion on Pharmacotherapy, 5(3), 691–698. https://doi.org/10.1517/14656566.5.3.691.

10   CDC. "Tetanus."

11   Amanna, I.J., and Slifka, M.K. "Duration of humoral immunity to common viral and vaccine antigens." New England Journal of Medicine, 357(19) (2007): 1903–1915.

12   Slifka AM, Park B, Gao L, Slifka MK. "Incidence of Tetanus and Diphtheria in Relation to Adult Vaccination Schedules." *Clin Infect Dis.* 2021 Jan 27;72(2):285–292. doi: 10.1093/cid/ciaa017. Erratum in: Clin Infect Dis. 2025 Feb 24;80(2):489. doi: 10.1093/cid/ciaf014. https://pubmed.ncbi.nlm.nih.gov/32095828/.

13   CDC. "Tetanus."

14   Ibid.

15   Ibid.

16   Ibid.

17   Humphries and Bystrianyk. "Dissolving Illusions."

18   Ibid.

19   US Bureau of Labor Statistics. "Employment by Major Industry Sector, 1947–2020." Accessed May 31, 2025.

20   CDC. "Tetanus."

21   Garbinsky D, Hunter S, La EM, Poston S, Hogea C. "State-Level Variations and Factors Associated with Adult Vaccination Coverage: A Multilevel Modeling Approach." *Pharmacoecon Open.* 2021 Sep;5(3):411–423. doi: 10.1007/s41669-021-00262-x. Epub 2021 Apr 16. PMID: 33860921; PMCID: PMC8333180.

22   Geier and Geier. "A review of the vaccine adverse event reporting system database."

23   Ibid.

24   Ibid.

Chapter 11

1   Informed Consent Action Network v. US Food and Drug Administration. (2019). Petition. Retrieved from https://icandecide.org/wp-content/uploads /2019/09/ICAvFDA-Resolved-Court-Filed-Copy.pdf.

2   Centers for Disease Control and Prevention. Pregnancy and vaccination. (Accessed July 16, 2025) https://www.cdc.gov/vaccines-pregnancy/about /index.html.

3   American College of Obstetricians and Gynecologists. (2025, May 26). ACOG statement on HHS recommendations regarding the COVID vaccine during pregnancy. https://www.acog.org/news/news-releases/2025/05/acog-statement -on-hhs-recommendations-regarding-the-covid-vaccine-during-pregnancy.

4   Brooks, J. T., & Butler, J. C. (2021). "Effectiveness of mask wearing to control community spread of SARS-CoV-2." *JAMA*, 325(10), 998–999. https: //doi.org/10.1001/jama.2021.1505.

5   Fineberg, H. V. (2017). "Pandemic preparedness and response—Lessons from the H1N1 influenza of 2009." *New England Journal of Medicine*, 370(14), 1335–1342. https://doi.org/10.1056/NEJMra1208802.

6   Institute of Medicine (US) Committee on the Effect of Climate Change on Indoor Air Quality and Public Health. (2011). "Climate change, the indoor environment, and health." *National Academies Press* (US). https://www.ncbi .nlm.nih.gov/books/NBK493173/.

7   Wu, S., Griffin, S. O., Edwards, C. M., & Jernigan, D. B. (2011). "Economic impact of the 2009 H1N1 influenza pandemic on the United States healthcare system." *Vaccine*, 29(47), 8583–8587. https://doi.org/10.1016/j. vaccine.2011.09.013.

8   Lee, B. Y., et al. (2013). "The economic burden of Clostridium difficile." *Clinical Microbiology and Infection*, 19(3), 217–223. https://doi.org/10.1111/j .1469–0691.2012.03868.x.

9   Li, Z., et al. (2021). "The role of long non-coding RNAs in the pathogenesis of hereditary diseases." *International Journal of Molecular Sciences*, 22(21), 11516. https://doi.org/10.3390/ijms222111516.

10   Keam, S. J., & Harper, J. E. (2014). "Emerging therapies for systemic lupus erythematosus—Focus on monoclonal antibodies." *Drug Design, Development and Therapy*, 8, 695–707. https://doi.org/10.2147/DDDT.S46062.

11   Wallace, D. J. (2016). *The lupus book: A guide for patients and their families* (5th ed.). Oxford University Press. https://pubmed.ncbi.nlm.nih.gov/27449682/.

12   Marks, K. J., et al. (2022). "Hospitalizations of children and adolescents with laboratory-confirmed COVID-19—COVID-NET, 14 states, March 1, 2020–February 26, 2022." *Morbidity and Mortality Weekly Report*, 71(10), 364–368. https://doi.org/10.15585/mmwr.mm7110a1.

13   Tartof, S. Y., et al. (2024). "Waning of 2-dose and 3-dose effectiveness of mRNA vaccines against COVID-19–associated emergency department and urgent care encounters and hospitalizations among adults during periods of Delta and Omicron variant predominance—VISION Network, 10 states, August 2021–January 2022." *The Journal of Infectious Diseases*, 229(4), 1151–1161. https://doi.org/10.1093/infdis/jiad542.

14   Shrestha, N. et al. "Effectiveness of the Influenza Vaccine During the 2024–2025 Respiratory Viral Season," *medRxiv* 2025.01.30.25321421; doi: https://doi.org/10.1101/2025.01.30.25321421.

15   Tostanoski, L. H., et al. (2023). "Durability of immune responses to mRNA booster vaccination against COVID-19." *The Journal of Infectious Diseases*, 227(12), 1433–1436. https://doi.org/10.1093/infdis/jiad054.

16   Ibid.

17   Navar-Boggan, A. M., et al. (2015). "Hyperlipidemia in early adulthood increases long-term risk of coronary heart disease." *Circulation*, 131(5), 451–458. https://doi.org/10.1161/CIRCULATIONAHA.114.012477.

18   Ibid.

19	Visher, E., et al. (2019). "The mutational robustness of influenza A virus." *Nature Communications*, 10, 3159. https://doi.org/10.1038/s41467–019-11296–5.

20	Fortune Business Insights. (2023). "Influenza vaccine market size, share & industry analysis, 2023–2030." https://www.fortunebusinessinsights.com /industry-reports/influenza-vaccine-market-101896.

21	McLean, H. Q., et al. (2023). "Influenza vaccine effectiveness against influenza A(H3N2)-related illness in the United States during the 2021–2022 influenza season." *Clinical Infectious Diseases*, 77(4), 578–587. https://doi .org/10.1093/cid/ciad139.

22	Centers for Disease Control and Prevention. (Accessed June 25, 2025). Pregnancy and vaccination. https://www.cdc.gov/vaccines-pregnancy/about/index.html.

23	American College of Obstetricians and Gynecologists. (2025, May 26). "ACOG statement on HHS recommendations regarding the COVID vaccine during pregnancy."

24	Bowden, P. A. (2023). "FOIA reveals troubling relationship between HHS/CDC & the American College of Obstetricians and Gynecologists." *America Out Loud News*. https://www.americaoutloud.news/foia-reveals -troubling-relationship-between-hhs-cdc-the-american-college-of-obstetricians -and-gynecologists/.

25	US Department of Health and Human Services. (2023). Community Corps. https://www.covid.gov/get-involved/community-corps.

26	CDC Foundation. (n.d.). Pregnant and protected: Vaccination during pregnancy. https://www.cdcfoundation.org/pregnant-and-protected.

27	Fast, H. E., et al. (2023). "Booster and additional primary dose COVID-19 vaccinations among adults aged ≥65 years—United States, August 13, 2021–November 19, 2022." Morbidity and Mortality Weekly Report, 72(46), 1257–1261. https://doi.org/10.15585/mmwr.mm7246a3.

28	Erman, M. (2022, January 7). "'Paramount importance': Judge orders FDA to hasten release of Pfizer vaccine docs." Reuters. https://www.reuters

.com/legal/government/paramount-importance-judge-orders-fda-hasten
-release-pfizer-vaccine-docs-2022–01-07/.

29   Wolf, N. (2022, April 29). "Bombshell: Pfizer and the FDA knew in early
     2021 that the Pfizer mRNA COVID vaccine caused dire fetal and infant
     risks. They began an aggressive campaign to vaccinate pregnant women
     anyway." *DailyClout*. https://dailyclout.io/bombshell-pfizer-and-the-fda
     -knew-in-early-2021-that-the-pfizer-mrna-covid-vaccine-caused-dire-fetal
     -and-infant-risks-they-began-an-aggressive-campaign-to-vaccinate-pregnant
     -women-anyway/.

30   Pfizer. (2021). Cumulative analysis of post-authorization adverse event
     reports of PF-07302048 (BNT162B2) received through 28-Feb-2021. Public
     Health and Medical Professionals for Transparency. https://www.phmpt
     .org/wp-content/uploads/2023/04/125742_S2_M1_pllr-cumulative-review
     .pdf.

31   Shimabukuro, T. T., et al. (2021). "Preliminary findings of mRNA COVID-
     19 vaccine safety in pregnant persons." *New England Journal of Medicine*,
     384(24), 2273–2282. https://doi.org/10.1056/NEJMoa2104983.

32   The HighWire with Del Bigtree. (2022, April 29). Naomi Wolf: Pfizer knew
     their vaccine would cause harm to babies [Video]. YouTube. https://www
     .youtube.com/watch?v=kbdoXen3AR8.

33   Gray, K. J., et al. (2021). "COVID-19 vaccine response in pregnant and lac-
     tating women: A cohort study." *American Journal of Obstetrics and Gynecology*,
     225(3), 303.e1–303.e17. https://doi.org/10.1016/j.ajog.2021.03.023.

34   Zauche, L. H., et al. (2021). "Receipt of mRNA COVID-19 vaccines and
     risk of spontaneous abortion." *New England Journal of Medicine*, 385(16),
     1533–1535. https://doi.org/10.1056/NEJMc2113516.

35   Lipkind, H. S., et al. (2022). "Receipt of COVID-19 vaccine during preg-
     nancy and preterm or small-for-gestational-age at birth—Eight integrated
     health care organizations, United States, December 15, 2020–July 22,

2021." *BJOG: An International Journal of Obstetrics & Gynaecology*, 129(12), 2064–2070. https://doi.org/10.1111/1471–0528.17721.

36   Guetzkow, J., Patalon, T., Gazit, S., Høeg, T. B., Fraiman, J., Segal, Y., & Levi, R. (2025). "Observed-to-expected fetal losses following mRNA COVID-19 vaccination in early pregnancy." medRxiv. https://doi.org/10.11 01/2025.06.18.25329352.

37   Manniche V, et al. "Rates of successful conceptions according to COVID-19 vaccination status: Data from the Czech Republic." *International Journal of Risk & Safety in Medicine.* 2025;0(0). doi:10.1177/09246479251353384.

38   Safford, H. C., Paul, M. R., & Mitchell, M. J. (2025). "Lipid nanoparticle-mediated mRNA delivery in pregnancy to prevent infectious disease-related fetal morbidity and mortality." Nano Letters. Advance online publication. https://mitchell-lab.seas.upenn.edu/wp-content/uploads/2025/04/Safford _NanoLetters.pdf.

39   Swingle K. L., et al. "Ionizable Lipid Nanoparticles for *In Vivo* mRNA Delivery to the Placenta during Pregnancy." *J Am Chem Soc.* 2023 Mar 1; 145(8):4691–4706. doi: 10.1021/jacs.2c12893.

40   Assessment report COVID-19 mRNA vaccine (nucleoside-modified). European Medicines 173 Agency (EMA). Procedure no. EMEA/H/C/005735 /0000. Accessed September 22, 2023. 174 Available at: https://www. ema.europa.eu/en/documents/assessment-report/comirnaty-epar-175 public-assessment-report_en.pdf.

41   Lin X, Botros B, Hanna M, Gurzenda E, Manzano De Mejia C, Chavez M, Hanna N, "Transplacental Transmission of the COVID-19 Vaccine mRNA: Evidence from Placental, Maternal and Cord Blood Analyses Post-Vaccination," *American Journal of Obstetrics and Gynecology* (2024), doi: https: //doi.org/10.1016/j.ajog.2024.01.022.

42   Lin X, Botros B, Hanna M, Gurzenda E, Manzano De Mejia C, Chavez M, Hanna N, "Transplacental Transmission of the COVID-19 Vaccine mRNA: Evidence from Placental, Maternal and Cord Blood Analyses

Post-Vaccination", *American Journal of Obstetrics and Gynecology* (2024), doi: https://doi.org/10.1016/j.ajog.2024.01.022.

43 Lioness of Judah Ministry. (2025, April 25). Absolutely devastating: Fibrous clots in the living linked to COVID-19 vaccination. Exposing The Darkness. https://lionessofjudah.substack.com/p/absolutely-devastating-fibrous-clots.

44 Atyabi SMH, et al. "Relationship between blood clots and COVID-19 vaccines: A literature review." *Open Life Sci.* 2022 Apr 26;17(1):401–415. doi: 10.1515/biol-2022–0035.

45 Chui CSL, et al. "Thromboembolic events and hemorrhagic stroke after mRNA (BNT162b2) and inactivated (CoronaVac) covid-19 vaccination: A self-controlled case series study." *EClinicalMedicine.* 2022 Jun 25;50:101504. doi: 10.1016/j.eclinm.2022.101504.

46 Rambaran RN, Serpell LC. "Amyloid fibrils: abnormal protein assembly." *Prion.* 2008 Jul-Sep;2(3):112–7. doi: 10.4161/pri.2.3.7488.

47 McCairn, K. W. (2025, May 30). "Amyloidogenic fibrils in a post-gestational case of mRNA vaccine exposure: Structural, pathophysiological, and biosecurity perspectives." Kevin W. McCairn Ph.D. https://kevinwmccairn phd282302.substack.com/p/amyloidogenic-fibrils-in-a-post-gestational.

48 Nyström, S. et al. "Amyloidogenesis of SARS-CoV-2 Spike Protein." *Journal of the American Chemical Society* **2022** *144* (20), 8945–8950 DOI: 10.1021/jacs.2c03925.

49 Pretorius E, Vlok M, Venter C, Bezuidenhout JA, Laubscher GJ, Steenkamp J, Kell DB. "Persistent clotting protein pathology in Long COVID/Post-Acute Sequelae of COVID-19 (PASC) is accompanied by increased levels of antiplasmin." *Cardiovasc Diabetol.* 2021 Aug 23;20(1):172. doi: 10.1186/s12933–021-01359–7.

50 Chudov, I. (2022, August 22). "How to make COVID vaccines appear safe for pregnant women." Igor's Newsletter. https://www.igor-chudov.com/p/how-to-make-covid-vaccines-appear.

51   Ibid.

52   Bookstein, F. L., et al. (2023). "Birth defects associated with COVID-19 vaccination in pregnancy: A cohort study in Sweden." *American Journal of Obstetrics and Gynecology*, 229(3), 245.e1–245.e11. https://doi.org/10.1016/j.ajog.2023.02.020.

53   Kharbanda, E. O., et al. (2023). "COVID-19 booster vaccination in early pregnancy and surveillance for spontaneous abortion." *JAMA Network Open*, 6(5), e2314350. https://doi.org/10.1001/jamanetworkopen.2023.14350.

54   Fell, D. B., et al. (2013). "Fetal death and preterm birth associated with maternal influenza vaccination: A systematic review." *Vaccine*, 31(45), 5168–5176. https://doi.org/10.1016/j.vaccine.2013.08.073.

55   Ibid.

56   Balgobin, C. A., & Economy, K. E. (2020). "Ischemic complications in pregnancy: Who is at risk?" *US Cardiology Review*, 14, e12. https://doi.org/10.15420/usc.2020.18.

57   Ciurica, S., et al. (2021). "Coronary artery disease in women: From diagnosis to treatment." Frontiers in Cardiovascular Medicine, 8, 646297. https://doi.org/10.3389/fcvm.2021.646297.

58   US Food and Drug Administration. (2018). FDA briefing document: Vaccines and Related Biological Products Advisory Committee meeting, September 19, 2018. https://www.fda.gov/media/119862/download.

59   US Food and Drug Administration. (2019). FDA briefing document: Vaccines and Related Biological Products Advisory Committee meeting, April 4, 2019. https://www.fda.gov/media/124002/download.

60   US Food and Drug Administration. (2022). FDA briefing document: Vaccines and Related Biological Products Advisory Committee meeting, January 26, 2022. https://www.fda.gov/media/162830/download.

61   US Food and Drug Administration. (2019). FDA briefing document: Vaccines and Related Biological Products Advisory Committee meeting, April 4, 2019. https://www.fda.gov/media/124002/download.

62   Fell, D. B., et al. (2013). "Influenza vaccination and fetal and neonatal outcomes." Expert Review of Vaccines, 12(12), 1417–1430. https://doi.org/10.1586/14760584.2013.851607.

63   Ciapponi, A., et al. (2023). "Influenza vaccines in immunosuppressed adults with cancer." Cochrane Database of Systematic Reviews, 2023(2), CD008983. https://doi.org/10.1002/14651858.CD008983.pub3.

64   US Food and Drug Administration. (2022). FDA briefing document: Vaccines and Related Biological Products Advisory Committee meeting, January 26, 2022. https://www.fda.gov/media/162830/download.

65   US Food and Drug Administration. (2019). FDA briefing document: Vaccines and Related Biological Products Advisory Committee meeting, April 4, 2019. https://www.fda.gov/media/124002/download.

66   Fleming-Dutra KE, Jones JM, Roper LE, et al. "Use of the Pfizer Respiratory Syncytial Virus Vaccine During Pregnancy for the Prevention of Respiratory Syncytial Virus–Associated Lower Respiratory Tract Disease in Infants: Recommendations of the Advisory Committee on Immunization Practices— United States, 2023." *MMWR Morb Mortal Wkly Rep* 2023;72:1115–1122. DOI: http://dx.doi.org/10.15585/mmwr.mm7241e1.

67   US Food and Drug Administration. (2023, August 21). FDA approves first vaccine for pregnant individuals to prevent RSV in infants. https://www.fda.gov/news-events/press-announcements/fda-approves-first-vaccine-pregnant-individuals-prevent-rsv-infants.

68   Centers for Disease Control and Prevention. (2024). Respiratory syncytial virus (RSV). https://www.cdc.gov/rsv/index.html.

69 Kampmann, B., et al. (2022). "Bivalent prefusion F vaccine in pregnancy to prevent RSV illness in infants." *New England Journal of Medicine*, 386(16), 1451–1460. https://doi.org/10.1056/NEJMoa2204670.

70 American College of Obstetricians and Gynecologists. (2023, September). Maternal respiratory syncytial virus vaccination. https://www.acog.org/clinical /clinical-guidance/practice-advisory/articles/2023/09/maternal-respiratory -syncytial-virus-vaccination APA Style (7th Edition).

71 Simões, E. A. F., et al. (2023). "Efficacy and safety of respiratory syncytial virus (RSV) prefusion F protein vaccine (RSVPreF3 OA) in older adults over 2 RSV seasons." *Clinical Infectious Diseases*, 76(7), 1153–1162. https: //doi.org/10.1093/cid/ciac920.

72 GlaxoSmithKline. (2022, February 22). "GSK provides further update on phase III RSV maternal vaccine candidate programme." https://www.gsk .com/en-gb/media/press-releases/gsk-provides-further-update-on-phase-iii -rsv-maternal-vaccine-candidate-programme.

73 US Food and Drug Administration. (2023). Vaccines and Related Biological Products Advisory Committee meeting, February 28–March 1, 2023: Briefing document. https://www.fda.gov/media/165621/download.

74 Madhi, S. A., et al. (2023). "Respiratory syncytial virus vaccination during pregnancy and effects in infants." *New England Journal of Medicine*, 389(16), 1463–1475. https://doi.org/10.1056/NEJMoa2304399.

75 Wise, J. (2023, November 7). "The BMJ investigates concerns over informed consent for pregnant women in Pfizer's trials." *BMJ*. https://www.bmj.com /company/newsroom/the-bmj-investigates-concerns-over-informed-consent -for-pregnant-women-in-pfizers-rsv-vaccine-trial/.

76 US Food and Drug Administration. (2023). Abrysvo (respiratory syncytial virus vaccine) prescribing information. https://www.fda.gov/media/168889 /download?attachment.

77 Ibid.

78 Fleming-Dutra KE, Jones JM, Roper LE, et al. "Use of the Pfizer Respiratory Syncytial Virus Vaccine During Pregnancy for the Prevention of Respiratory Syncytial Virus–Associated Lower Respiratory Tract Disease in Infants: Recommendations of the Advisory Committee on Immunization Practices— United States, 2023." *MMWR Morb Mortal Wkly Rep* 2023;72:1115–1122. DOI: http://dx.doi.org/10.15585/mmwr.mm7241e1.

79 World Health Organization. (2023, May 10). Preterm birth. https://www.who.int/news-room/fact-sheets/detail/preterm-birth.

80 Goldenberg, R. L., et al. (2016). "The preterm birth syndrome: Issues to consider in creating a classification system." *American Journal of Obstetrics and Gynecology*, 215(2), 141–149. https://doi.org/10.1016/j.ajog.2016.02.030.

81 Vogel, J. P., et al. (2020). "The global epidemiology of preterm birth." *Best Practice & Research Clinical Obstetrics & Gynaecology*, 67, 3–12. https://doi.org/10.1016/j.bpobgyn.2020.04.003.

82 Centers for Disease Control and Prevention. (2023, May 31). Jaundice facts. https://www.cdc.gov/ncbddd/jaundice/facts.html.

83 Eunice Kennedy Shriver National Institute of Child Health and Human Development. (2022, January 31). "What are the risks of preeclampsia & eclampsia to the mother?" https://www.nichd.nih.gov/health/topics/preeclampsia/conditioninfo/risk-mother.

84 Dimitriadis, E., et al. (2023). "Pre-eclampsia." *Nature Reviews Disease Primers*, 9(1), 8. https://doi.org/10.1038/s41572-023-00417-6.

85 Magee, L. A., et al. (2021). "The 2021 International Society for the Study of Hypertension in Pregnancy classification, diagnosis & management recommendations for international practice." *Pregnancy Hypertension*, 27, 148–169. https://doi.org/10.1016/j.preghy.2021.09.008.

86 Ibid.

87 US Food and Drug Administration. (2025, January 7). FDA requires Guillain-Barré syndrome (GBS) warning in the prescribing information

for RSV vaccines Abrysvo and Arexvy. https://www.fda.gov/vaccines-blood
-biologics/safety-availability-biologics/fda-requires-guillain-barre-syndrome
-gbs-warning-prescribing-information-rsv-vaccines-abrysvo-and.

88   Ibid.

Chapter 12

1   Carlson, Robert H. "HPV Vaccine, Now FDA-Approved, Shown to Protect
     against Vaginal, Vulvar Intraepithelial Neoplasias." *Oncology Times* Supplement
     (August 2006): 2–4. https://doi.org/10.1097/01.cot.0000316086.11194.af.

2   "HPV Vaccine." Centers for Disease Control and Prevention, August 16,
     2023. https://www.cdc.gov/hpv/parents/vaccine-for-hpv.html.

3   Ibid.

4   Luria, Lynette, and Gabriella Cardoza-Favarato. StatPearls [Internet].
     Treasure Island, FL: StatPearls Publishing, 2024.

5   Anna Szymonowicz. "Biological and Clinical Aspects of HPV-Related
     Cancers." *Cancer Biology and Medicine* 17, no. 4 (2020): 864–78. https://doi
     .org/10.20892/j.issn.2095–3941.2020.0370.

6   Erkinovich, et al. "HPV—Relevance, Oncogenesis and Diagnosis (A
     Review)". *European Journal of Innovation in Nonformal Education* 3, no. 1
     (2023):129–34. https://www.inovatus.es/index.php/ejine/article/view/1426.

7   "HPV and Cancer." National Cancer Institute. Accessed January 25, 2024.
     https://www.cancer.gov/about-cancer/causes-prevention/risk/infectious-agents
     /hpv-and-cancer.

8   Ibid.

9   Ibid.

10   "HPV-Associated Cancer Diagnosis by Age." Centers for Disease Control
     and Prevention, September 12, 2023. https://www.cdc.gov/cancer/hpv
     /statistics/age.htm.

11 Arbyn, Marc, Elisabete Weiderpass, Laia Bruni, Silvia de Sanjosé, Mona Saraiya, Jacques Ferlay, and Freddie Bray. "Estimates of Incidence and Mortality of Cervical Cancer in 2018: A Worldwide Analysis." *The Lancet Global Health* 8, no. 2 (February 2020). https://doi.org/10.1016/s2214-109x(19)30482-6.

12 Ibid.

13 "Cancer of the Cervix Uteri—Cancer Stat Facts." SEER. Accessed January 25, 2024. https://seer.cancer.gov/statfacts/html/cervix.html.

14 The Future II Study Group. "Quadrivalent Vaccine against Human Papillomavirus to Prevent High-Grade Cervical Lesions." *New England Journal of Medicine* 356, no. 19 (May 10, 2007): 1915–27. https://doi .org/10.1056/nejmoa061741.

15 Merck Sharp & Dohme LLC. *GARDASIL.* Food and Drug Administration. April, 2023. https://www.fda.gov/media/90064/download?attachment.

16 Vink, M., et al. "Clinical Progression of High- Grade Cervical Intraepithelial Neoplasia: Estimating the Time to Preclinical Cervical Cancer from Doubly Censored National Registry Data." *American Journal of Epidemiology* 178, no. 7 (July 28, 2013): 1161–69. https://doi.org/10.1093/aje/kwt077.

17 Burnett, Tatnai. "Do Atypical Cells Usually Mean Cancer?" Mayo Clinic, September 16, 2022. https://www.mayoclinic.org/diseases-conditions/cancer /expert-answers/atypical-cells/faq-20058493.

18 Vink, M. et al. "Clinical Progression of High-Grade Cervical Intraepithelial Neoplasia: Estimating the Time to Preclinical Cervical Cancer from Doubly Censored National Registry Data." *American Journal of Epidemiology* 178, no. 7 (July 28, 2013): 1161–69. https://doi.org/10.1093/aje/kwt077.

19 "Abnormal Pap Smear Follow-Up." Roswell Park Comprehensive Cancer Center. Accessed January 25, 2024. https://www.roswellpark.org/cancer talk/201811/abnormal-pap-smear-follow.

20   Baden, Lindsey R., Gregory D. Curfman, Stephen Morrissey, and Jeffrey M. Drazen. "Human Papillomavirus Vaccine—Opportunity and Challenge." *New England Journal of Medicine* 356, no. 19 (May 10, 2007): 1990–91. https://doi.org/10.1056/nejme078088.

21   Slade, Barbara A. "Postlicensure Safety Surveillance for Quadrivalent Human Papillomavirus Recombinant Vaccine." *JAMA* 302, no. 7 (August 19, 2009): 750. https://doi.org/10.1001/jama.2009.1201.

22   Ibid.

23   "HPV Vaccine Safety and Effectiveness." Centers for Disease Control and Prevention, November 16, 2021. https://www.cdc.gov/vaccines/vpd/hpv/hcp/safety-effectiveness.html.

24   Ibid.

25   Ibid.

26   Merck Sharp & Dohme LLC. *GARDASIL*. Food and Drug Administration. April, 2023. https://www.fda.gov/media/90064/download?attachment.

27   Hviid, A., H. Svanström, N. M. Scheller, O. Grönlund, B. Pasternak, and L. Arnheim-Dahlström. "Human Papillomavirus Vaccination of Adult Women and Risk of Autoimmune and Neurological Diseases." *Journal of Internal Medicine* 283, no. 2 (October 18, 2017): 154–65. https://doi.org/10.1111/joim.12694.

28   Little, Deirdre Therese, and Harvey Rodrick Ward. "Adolescent Premature Ovarian Insufficiency Following Human Papillomavirus Vaccination." *Journal of Investigative Medicine High Impact Case Reports* 2, no. 4 (October 1, 2014) https://doi.org/10.1177/2324709614556129.

29   Segal, Yahel, and Yehuda Shoenfeld. "Vaccine-Induced Autoimmunity: The Role of Molecular Mimicry and Immune Crossreaction." *Cellular & Molecular Immunology* 15, no. 6 (March 5, 2018): 586–94. https://doi.org/10.1038/cmi.2017.151.

30 Ivette Maldonado, Nicolas Rodríguez Niño, et al. "Evaluation of the safety profile of the quadrivalent vaccine against human papillomavirus in the risk of developing autoimmune, neurological, and hematological diseases in adolescent women in Colombia." *Vaccine.* Published online. (March 7, 2024). https://www.sciencedirect.com/science/article/pii/S0264410X24002639. Merck Sharp & Dohme LLC. *GARDASIL.* Food and Drug Administration. April, 2023. https://www.fda.gov/media/90064/download?attachment.

31 Wastila, L., Fu, Y.-H., Tung, C.-C., et al. (2025). "Association between vaccination for human papillomavirus (HPV) and autonomic dysfunction and menstrual irregularities: A self-controlled case series analysis." Drugs—Real World Outcomes. https://doi.org/10.1007/s40801-025-00504-y.

32 Merck Sharp & Dohme LLC. *GARDASIL.* Food and Drug Administration. April, 2023. https://www.fda.gov/media/90064/download?attachment.

33 Ibid.

34 Martínez-Lavín, Manuel. "HPV Vaccination Syndrome: A Clinical Mirage, or a New Tragic Fibromyalgia Model." *Reumatología Clínica* (English Edition) 14, no. 4 (July 2018): 211–14. https://doi.org/10.1016/j.reumae.2018.01.001.

35 Merck Sharp & Dohme LLC. *GARDASIL.* Food and Drug Administration. April, 2023. https://www.fda.gov/media/90064/download?attachment.

36 Shaw, Christopher A., and Michael S. Petrik. "Aluminum Hydroxide Injections Lead to Motor Deficits and Motor Neuron Degeneration." *Journal of Inorganic Biochemistry* 103, no. 11 (November 2009): 1555–62. https://doi.org/10.1016/j.jinorgbio.2009.05.019.

37 Shaw, C. A., and L. Tomljenovic. "Aluminum in the Central Nervous System (CNS): Toxicity in Humans and Animals, Vaccine Adjuvants, and Autoimmunity." *Immunologic Research* 56, no. 2–3 (April 23, 2013): 304–16. https://doi.org/10.1007/s12026-013-8403-1. https://www.nature.com/articles/s41598-020-64734-6

38 Exley, Christopher, and Elizabeth Clarkson. "Aluminium in Human Brain Tissue from Donors without Neurodegenerative Disease: A Comparison with Alzheimer's Disease, Multiple Sclerosis and Autism." *Scientific Reports* 10, no. 1 (May 8, 2020). https://doi.org/10.1038/s41598–020-64734–6.

39 Mehlsen, Jesper, Louise Brinth, Kirsten Pors, Kim Varming, Gerd Wallukat, and Rikke Katrine Olsen. "Autoimmunity in Patients Reporting Long-Term Complications after Exposure to Human Papilloma Virus Vaccination." *Journal of Autoimmunity* 133 (December 2022): 102921. https://doi.org/10.1016/j .jaut.2022.102921.

40 Ibid.

41 Ibid. https://www.ncbi.nlm.nih.gov/pmc/articles/PMC2278297/.

42 Lippman, Abby, Madeline Boscoe, and Carol Scurfield. "Do you approve of spending $300 million on HPV vaccination?: No." Canadian family physician, Medecin de famille canadien, 54, no. 2, (2008) 175–181. https://www .ncbi.nlm.nih.gov/pmc/articles/PMC2278297/.

43 "List of grants for research to increase uptake of HPV vaccines." Children's Health Defense. Accessed January 26, 2024. https://childrenshealthdefense .org/wp-content/uploads/02–20-2020-Facts-about-HPV.pdf.

44 "Gavi Board Meeting, 7–8 December 2022." Gavi, The Vaccine Alliance. December, 2022. Accessed January 25, 2024. https://www.gavi.org /governance/gavi-board/minutes/7–8-december-2022

45 "About Our Alliance." Gavi, The Vaccine Alliance. Accessed January 25, 2024. https://www.gavi.org/our-alliance/about.

46 Pharmacovigilance Risk Assessment Committee (PRAC). "Assessment Report: Human Papillomavirus (HPV) Vaccines," November 11, 2015. https://www .ema.europa.eu/en/documents/referral/hpv-vaccines-article-20-procedure -assessment-report_en.pdf.

47 Ibid. https://www.ncbi.nlm.nih.gov/pmc/articles/PMC9762824/.

48   Abouelella DK, et al. "Human papillomavirus vaccine uptake among teens before and during the COVID-19 pandemic in the United States." *Hum Vaccin Immunother.* 2022 Dec 30;18(7):2148825. doi: 10.1080/21645515 .2022.2148825.

49   Suk, Ryan, Kaiping Liao, Cici X. Bauer, Catherine Basil, and Meng Li. "Human Papillomavirus Vaccine Administration Trends among Commercially Insured US Adults Aged 27–45 Years before and after Advisory Committee on Immunization Practices Recommendation Change, 2007–2020." *JAMA Health Forum* 3, no. 12 (December 16, 2022). https: //doi.org/10.1001/jamahealthforum.2022.4716.

50   VRBPAC. "VRBPAC Background Document Gardasil™ HPV Quadrivalent Vaccine May 18, 2006 VRBPAC Meeting." *Zenodo*, May 18, 2006. https: //doi.org/10.5281/zenodo.1434214.

51   Dunne, Eileen F., Elizabeth R. Unger, Maya Sternberg, Geraldine McQuillan, David C. Swan, Sonya S. Patel, and Lauri E. Markowitz. "Prevalence of HPV Infection among Females in the United States." *JAMA* 297, no. 8 (February 28, 2007): 813. https://doi.org/10.1001/jama.297.8.813.Slade, Barbara A. "Postlicensure Safety Surveillance for Quadrivalent Human Papillomavirus Recombinant Vaccine." *JAMA* 302, no. 7 (August 19, 2009): 750. https://doi .org/10.1001/jama.2009.1201.

52   Slade, Barbara A. "Postlicensure Safety Surveillance for Quadrivalent Human Papillomavirus Recombinant Vaccine." *JAMA* 302, no. 7 (August 19, 2009): 750. https://doi.org/10.1001/jama.2009.1201.

53   Ibid.

54   Ibid.

55   Tomljenovic, Lucija, Emily Tarsell, James Garrett, Christopher A. Shaw, and Mary S. Holland. "Significant Under-Reporting of Quadrivalent Human Papillomavirus Vaccine-Associated Serious Adverse Events in the United States: Time for Change? *Science, Public Health Policy, and The Law.*

2 (May 2021):37–58. https://cf5e727d-d029fe2d3ad957f.filesusr.com/ugd /adf864_2dede593f4a04e64ab6c0c45bc14d450.pdf.

56 Ibid.

57 US Food and Drug Administration. "CFR—Code of Federal Regulations Title 21." October 17, 2023. https://www.accessdata.fda.gov/scripts/cdrh/ cfdocs/cfcfr/cfrsearch.cfm?fr=312.32#. "Cancer of the Cervix Uteri— Cancer Stat Facts." SEER. Accessed January 25, 2024. https://seer.cancer .gov/statfacts/html/cervix.html.

58 "Cancer of the Cervix Uteri—Cancer Stat Facts." SEER. Accessed January 25, 2024. https://seer.cancer.gov/statfacts/html/cervix.html.

59 Ibid.

60 Issanov, Alpamys, Mohammad Karim, Gulzhanat Aimagambetova, and Trevor Dummer. "Does Vaccination Protect against Human Papillomavirus-Related Cancers? Preliminary Findings from the United States National Health and Nutrition Examination Survey (2011–2018)." Vaccines 10, no. 12 (December 10, 2022): 2113. https://doi.org/10.3390/vaccines10122113.

61 Ibid.

62 Hartman, Melissa. "Cervical Cancer Is Preventable." Johns Hopkins Bloomberg School of Public Health, January 24, 2023. https://public health.jhu.edu/2023/cervical-cancer-is-preventable. https://jamanetwork.com /journals/jama/fullarticle/2697704; Huang, Yu, Xinzhi Wu, Ying Lin, Wenzhou Li, Jiahua Liu, and Baozhi Song. "Multiple Sexual Partners and Vaginal Microecological Disorder Are Associated with HPV Infection and Cervical Carcinoma Development." Oncology Letters 20, no. 2 (June 16, 2020): 1915–21. https://doi.org/10.3892/ol.2020.11738.

63 US Preventive Services Task Force. Screening for Cervical Cancer: US Preventive Services Task Force Recommendation Statement. JAMA. 2018;320(7):674–686. doi:10.1001/jama.2018.10897

64 Ibid.

65 Huang, Yu, Xinzhi Wu, Ying Lin, Wenzhou Li, Jiahua Liu, and Baozhi Song. "Multiple Sexual Partners and Vaginal Microecological Disorder Are Associated with HPV Infection and Cervical Carcinoma Development." *Oncology Letters* 20, no. 2 (June 16, 2020): 1915–21. https://doi.org/10.3892/ol.2020.11738.

66 "How Do Viruses Mutate and What It Means for a Vaccine?" Pfizer. 2024. https://www.pfizer.com/news/articles/how_do_viruses_mutate_and_what_it_means_for_a_vaccine.

67 Ibid.

68 Fischer, S., Bettstetter, M., Becher, A., Lessel, M., Bank, C., Krams, M. . . . Gaumann, A. (2016). "Shift in prevalence of HPV types in cervical cytology specimens in the era of HPV vaccination." *Oncology Letters,* 12, 601–610. https://doi.org/10.3892/ol.2016.4668.

69 Ibid.

70 Ibid.

71 Guo, Fangjian, Jacqueline M. Hirth, and Abbey B. Berenson. "Human Papillomavirus Vaccination and Pap Smear Uptake among Young Women in the United States: Role of Provider and Patient." *Journal of Women's Health* 26, no. 10 (October 2017): 1114–22. https://doi.org/10.1089/jwh.2017.6424.

Chapter 13

1 Children's Health Defense. "Read the Fine Print: Vaccine Package Inserts Reveal Hundreds of Medical Conditions Linked to Vaccines." Children's Health Defense, 29 Apr. 2020. https://childrenshealthdefense.org/news/read-the-fine-print-vaccine-package-inserts-reveal-hundreds-of-medical-conditions-linked-to-vaccines/.

2 Ibid.

3 Ibid.

4   Ibid.

5   Merck & Co., Inc. AquaMEPHYTON (Phytonadione Injectable Emulsion, USP) [Package Insert]. US Food and Drug Administration, Mar. 2018. https://www.accessdata.fda.gov/drugsatfda_docs/label/2018/012223s041lbl.pdf.

Chapter 14

1   National Commission for the Protection of Human Subjects of Biomedical and Behavioral Research. (1979). The Belmont Report: Ethical principles and guidelines for the protection of human subjects of research. US Department of Health and Human Services. https://www.hhs.gov/ohrp/regulations-and-policy/belmont-report/read-the-belmont-report/index.html.

2   Ibid.

3   WKYC. (2021, October 11). Organ transplant surgery canceled due to new Cleveland Clinic policy requiring COVID-19 vaccination. https://www.wkyc.com/article/news/local/lake-county/organ-transplant-surgery-canceled-new-cleveland-clinic-policy-requiring-covid-19-vaccination/95–6dbf87d1-a246–46dd-8575–7d0ff1451a2a).

4   McCullough, P. A. (2020, November 19). Early outpatient treatment: An essential part of a COVID-19 solution [Testimony before the US Senate Committee on Homeland Security and Governmental Affairs]. US Senate Committee on Homeland Security and Governmental Affairs. https://www.hsgac.senate.gov/wp-content/uploads/imo/media/doc/Testimony-McCullough-2020–11-19.pdf.

5   World Health Organization. (n.d.). Module 1: Introduction to therapeutics for COVID-19. https://www.who.int/docs/default-source/coronaviruse/module-1-introduction-to-therapeutics-for-covid-19.pdf.

6   Publix Super Markets, Inc. (n.d.). Pharmacy services: Vaccines. Publix.com. https://www.publix.com/pharmacy/pharmacy-services/vaccines?searchterm redirect=immunization.

7   Nevada County, California. (2024, May 9). Immunization consent form
     (English). https://www.nevadacountyca.gov/DocumentCenter/View/53935/IZ
     -Consent-Form-English-5924---Fillable?bidId=.

8   Rite Aid Corporation. (2021, February 10). Immunization consent form
     (English). https://www.riteaid.com/content/dam/riteaid-web/pharmacy/vaccine
     -central/immunization-information/Immunization_Form_UPDATE_
     ENGLISH_FINAL-210210.pdf.

Chapter 15

1   https://www.cnbc.com/2021/12/01/how-hiv-research-paved-the-way-for
     -the-covid-mrna-vaccines.html?&qsearchterm=HIV%20research.

2   Johns Hopkins Medicine. (2018, May 31). "Infection rates after colonos-
     copy, endoscopy at US specialty centers are far higher than previously
     thought." https://www.hopkinsmedicine.org/news/newsroom/news-releases
     /2018/05/infection-rates-after-colonoscopy-endoscopy-at-us-specialty-centers
     -are-far-higher-than-previously-thought.

3   Giess, C. S., et al. (2018). "Complications of Breast Biopsy: A Review."
     American Journal of Roentgenology, 211(3), W139–W145. DOI: 10.2214/
     AJR.18.19723.

4   Manchikanti, L., et al. (2016). "Safety of Epidural Corticosteroid Injections."
     Drugs R&D, 16(1), 19–34. DOI: 10.1007/s40268–015-0119–3.

5   Adult Vaccines Now. (n.d.). CDC Releases Data Showing Safety of COVID
     Vaccines. Alliance for Aging Research. https://adultvaccinesnow.org/resources
     /cdc-releases-data-showing-safety-of-covid-vaccines/ (accessed July 9, 2025).

6   Junchao Li, et al. Post-licensure safety of respiratory syncytial virus vac-
     cines, Vaccine Adverse Event Reporting System, United States, May 2023–
     December 2024. Preventive Medicine Reports, Volume 56, 2025. https://
     doi.org/10.1016/j.pmedr.2025.103150.

7   Walach, H. Covid-19 vaccinations, self-reported health, and worldviews –
     A representative survey from Germany. Medical Research Archives, v. 12,
     n. 12, Dec. 2024. ISSN 2375–1924. https://esmed.org/MRA/mra/article
     /view/6205.

8   Kaiser Family Foundation. (2025, January 28). "Poll: Trust in public
     health agencies and vaccines falls amid Republican skepticism." KFF Health
     Information and Trust. https://www.kff.org/health-information-trust/press
     -release/poll-trust-in-public-health-agencies-and-vaccines-falls-amid-republican
     -skepticism/[](https://www.kff.org/health-information-and-trust/press-release
     /poll-trust-in-public-health-agencies-and-vaccines-falls-amid-republican
     -skepticism/)

Index